Everything You Need For
The 5:2 Diet

Polly Fielding   Lucy Lonsdale   Emily Hanson

ISBN-13:978-1497423206
ISBN-10:1497423201

This book is dedicated to everyone on the 5:2 diet.

We wish you the same success we've enjoyed.

CONTENTS

Introduction

By buying this book you have taken the first step to becoming the person you want to be. Within a short space of time, you will be amazed to see great results, with very little effort on your part.

The 5:2 diet is far from being a faddy one. In fact it's not so much a diet as a completely different view of what, when and how we eat. It's a whole new approach to food that is extremely effective and satisfying. You will finally be in control of your eating patterns and you'll find food so much more enjoyable without any guilt attached to enjoying your favourite treats.

Who are we?

We are three friends who were desperate to lose weight, trying any and practically every diet out there. Polly was the first of us to follow the 5:2 diet. Her passion for it inspired Lucy to begin. And, after a few months of watching the effect it had on their lives, Emily was finally persuaded to take the plunge.

As well as cajoling and encouraging each other along the way, we enthusiastically shared our ideas. At last we had found an eating pattern that really worked for us and involved very little willpower, which is just what we had been looking for!

After tackling the 5:2 diet in our individual ways, we decided to collaborate in producing a book with a comprehensive explanation of how and why this method of eating is so successful. We've pooled all our research and resources: in addition to recounting our personal experiences of the diet, we have included 135 recipes, plans for 72 meals, a section on mindful eating, a calorie counter and a calorie chart. We've designed the book to give you as much flexibility and choice as you could possibly want.

A brief note for American readers

According to the writer George Bernard Shaw, the British and Americans are two nations *divided* by a common language. We're aware, for instance that the wispy green leaf we call 'rocket', you call 'arugula'. Similarly, our 'courgette' is your 'zucchini', a name you borrowed from the Italians, whereas we copied the French. Whilst we've tried to keep this in mind and hope everything makes intelligent and intelligible sense to you, we hope also that you will be tolerant of any uniquely British words or expressions – to say nothing of the spellings - that may have crept in. They weren't intended to confuse you, really they weren't!

If a couple of the brand names do not exist in the USA, we're sure you will find plenty of suitable alternatives in your local grocery store. The calorie count is the important factor!

In the UK nowadays, metric measurements have become as commonplace as Imperial ones, possibly even more so. We've done conversions for you to make life easier, but you may still be interested to know that 28 grams are equal to one ounce (so 56 grams are 2 oz, 84 grams are 3 oz...) and that 1 fluid ounce equals 29.6 milliliters (ml) which is as close to 30ml as makes no difference (the remaining 0.4ml would be the drop that makes a tiny stain on your sweater!).

Chapter 1

Weighing Up The 5:2 Diet

What is the 5:2 Diet?

Put very simply, it's a way of eating that involves choosing any two days each week and restricting your total calorie intake on those days to no more than 500 calories for women or 600 for men. For the other five days you can follow your normal diet.

How does this diet differ from any other one out there?

It differs in that you have only to follow it for two days a week, unlike other diets which entail changing the way you eat on a daily basis. It does not make you envious of someone who is tucking in to your favourite high fat, calorie-laden foods, since you know that on the other five days you also have that choice. And, as well as losing weight, there are other health benefits and good reasons to adopt this intermittent form of calorie restriction.

What are the benefits of the 5:2 Diet?

Steady weight loss, which is virtually guaranteed if you are following this diet, is only one of the advantages even though it is clearly an important one and the one that attracts most people to it in the first place. But research strongly suggests that it also protects against developing some brain diseases such as Alzheimer's and Parkinson's. In addition, it can lower unhealthy cholesterol levels, normalize blood glucose, raise your energy levels and help you to live longer. And if those are not sufficient reasons to give it a try, it is worth considering the claim that this diet also affords protection from developing heart disease, type 2 diabetes and cancer.

That sounds impressive, but what evidence is there that this diet really does have these benefits?

There has been great deal of research with rodents and studies with humans are becoming more numerous. The Institute of Aging, in Baltimore, Maryland, USA, conducted controlled studies with mice that showed definitively that the ones who were fed the 5:2 way lived longer in mice years than the group who were fed normally. They also showed a far slower decline in brain function than the other mice. Additionally, they appeared more energetic and active than their fellow mice and displayed a markedly lower tendency to develop the sort of other diseases mentioned above. Whilst all this is very promising we cannot be certain that human beings will respond in precisely the same way.

However, we don't want to give the impression that we are anything less than enthusiastic about this diet which many people are finding very helpful. Research with the mice is a useful indicator that for most of us, this diet could well prove to be the best way forward for eating our way to considerably longer, healthier lives.

Only long term scientifically reliable, controlled studies with a significant number of people will give us the answers we seek. For the time being there is an enormous amount of anecdotal evidence from people who have successfully stayed on the 5:2 diet for several months or even longer. So we have enough information already to make our own informed decision about embarking on this diet; and our own experience will tell us if it suits us.

I have heard Laron Syndrome mentioned in connection with the 5:2 Diet. What is it?

In a village in Ecuador there is a group of around a hundred villagers who have Laron Syndrome (named after Zvi Laron, an Israeli researcher who first reported this condition in the nineteen sixties). They have been scientifically studied over a period of twenty-two years to find out why, barring alcoholism and accidents, they were living much longer lives than any of the other villagers. The reason seems to be that they have a genetic lack of the IGF-1 growth hormone which is responsible for childhood growth. This hormone lack accounts for why people in this group are unusually small - mostly less than three and a half feet tall.

So unusual and rare is the syndrome worldwide (affecting about three hundred people in total) that it has attracted much interest from scientists who have studied the villagers and others with this condition and then applied their findings to animal research.

Those with Laron Syndrome in the Ecuadorian village do not diet, some smoke and they all eat whatever food they want. Yet despite leading what we might consider very unhealthy lives and some becoming obese, they do not develop many of the usual serious illnesses like diabetes, cancer, heart disease and onset of brain diseases such as dementia, associated with age. They also look much younger for longer and generally live to a greater age than those without this syndrome. If they ate more healthily and did not smoke they would probably live even longer but knowing that they have this immunity tends to make them carefree rather than focus on living a hundred years or more.

Ok, but what has this got to do with the 5:2 diet specifically?

It has been discovered that the IGF-1 hormone, essential whilst we are growing into adults, can work against us once we begin to age. High amounts of it appear to cause damage to cells, which leads to a greater susceptibility to developing serious health problems. This in turn lowers our quality of life as well as shortening it considerably. Restricting calorie intake on the two days a week, as in the 5:2 diet, causes a lowering of the level of the insulin-like IGF-1 hormone, kick-starting our bodies into switching on DNA repair genes and focusing on the essential reparation of existing damaged cells instead of making new ones.

Following this diet is a brilliant way to ensure that our bodies can begin to undo the harm already done to cells and reverse some potentially serious effects of the aging process.

Is this a totally new concept?

Not at all. Way back in time our ancestors did not have three meals a day, fast food outlets or a great choice of supermarkets. They had to go out and hunt for food. So on some days they ate a feast, whilst on other days they ate very little unless they were exceptionally clever hunters with a lot of slow running animals nearby! Then, as time passed, people grew a lot of their food which meant that it wasn't plentiful all the time because it was seasonal. Later still, during World War Two and for some years after, food was rationed. Obesity was not a problem. It can't just be co-incidence that a large proportion of the UK population (post war baby boomers) are still alive and kicking! They were brought up on fresh food - many homes did not own a refrigerator until the fifties so meat, fruit and vegetables had to be bought daily or kept in a large cupboard, better known as a larder, for a few days.

Well, that's the history lesson over!

This sounds good so far but is it a safe diet to follow?

I have consulted a number of medical doctors about this and all of them say that, as long as the diet is followed sensibly (not becoming obsessive over calorie-counting, keeping it to two days per week and eating a normal diet on the other five days), it cannot harm, and could possibly be very beneficial. Some of them have, in fact, started this diet themselves!

Are there any reasons why anyone should not go on this diet?

Yes, it is definitely not suitable for children, pregnant or breast-feeding women, diabetics, or someone with an eating disorder. Furthermore, if you have any serious health problem or are in doubt about whether this form of eating is suitable for you, it is very important that you consult your GP before making a decision.

If I develop a medical problem whilst on this program, should I discontinue it?

Anyone with a health issue needs to consult their doctor before continuing *any* weight-loss program.

If I feel unwell is it still OK to pursue my low-calorie intake on that day?

On balance, it is best to wait until you feel better. Just choose a different day. One of the good things about this diet is that you can change your days around to suit your needs. You have total control.

Some nutritionists have expressed worries that food restriction carries a danger of developing eating disorders. Could this happen?

Being obsessive about any form of dieting can trigger an eating disorder. As far as the 5:2 diet is concerned, 'starvation' and 'fasting' are words that have been used by some to describe the two days of calorie restriction. If these terms are taken literally (i.e. no food whatsoever) then someone could develop anorexia, especially if they then began also to severely restrict their calorie intake for the rest of the week. Likewise, it is possible to become bulimic if, after each low calorie day, a person starts binge eating.

It's really about taking a sensible approach and not allowing food (or the lack of it) to become the central focus of your entire life.

The 5:2 diet carries an extremely low risk for most people of becoming eating-disordered, probably less so than in the case of many other, more faddish diets. That is, of course, provided it is tackled with a large dose of common sense and does not totally exclude any important groups of food that our bodies need. A particular advantage of this form of eating is that no food is completely banned.

But isn't binge eating a realistic possibility the day after consuming only a quarter of the normal daily calorie amount?

On the face of it you would think that this could well happen. It's understandable to assume that restricting calorie intake on one day would lead to gorging on food the next. However, we are creatures of habit and, surprising as it might seem, tend to revert to our normal eating patterns. This has certainly been the case for the majority on this diet. Indeed, after a few weeks most people have found that their appetite actually decreases. Even the scientists who have closely observed 5:2 dieters have been surprised by this fact.

It's not difficult to start a diet with enthusiasm but how easy is it to stick to this one?

We have spoken to many people who have had experience of trying out lots of diets – 'The cabbage soup diet', 'The Atkins diet', 'The morning banana diet' are a few that randomly spring to mind. Results with some of these were initially encouraging, with impressive weight loss whilst on them. But will power is a tricky thing and for all but a rare handful of mortals, persevering for a lengthy period with any regime that permanently denies them their favourite foods is too difficult.

With the 5:2 diet, on the other hand, you do not have to cut out any of the foods you like. Even if their calorie count is way too high to include in the low calorie days, you can enjoy them on the other five days of the week. This is probably the main reason that this particular diet is becoming so widespread. Many have started and, months later, are still on it. It's not a fad diet but rather a different way of eating. Not only do people on it see results quickly but they know that, even if they are finding it hard going, they have five other days a week when they eat normally and with less sense of guilt than previously.

It does not become unmanageable when you only have to think about reducing your calories for two days in a week instead of struggling with cutting them down every single day! And since you decide which two days in the week are best for you as well as being able to alter them week by week according to your social schedule (you probably won't want to choose any day you're going out to a restaurant, for example), the choice is all yours. Each week may have a different two days or you may find it more convenient to keep to the same two.

Should my lower-calorie days be consecutive or non-consecutive?

This is entirely up to you. If you wish to leave a few days in between, that's fine. If it suits you better to do consecutive days each week, no problem. It very much depends on your lifestyle.

How much weight will I actually lose a week?

There is no hard and fast answer to this, although you *will* lose weight if you are following the diet as we have outlined. A broad average is around 2 - 3 pounds a week. Some weeks you may lose more, some weeks a bit less. It's the overall weight loss that's important in the long term.

How often should I weigh myself?

It is important not to become obsessive about jumping on the scales. Once a week is quite sufficient to monitor your progress. It is a good idea to weigh yourself first thing in the morning (You might beneficially do this the day after your second reduced-calorie day in the week).

What if I finally find my weight is beginning to drop further than I wanted. Is that the time to stop?

No, because if you reach that stage you can simply drop to having one low calorie day per week to maintain your current healthy weight.

I enjoy cooking but on my low calorie days will I have to eat plain, boring foods and only a small amount of those?

On the contrary, as the recipes in this book will demonstrate, you can have fun producing a good variety of colourful, interesting meals to suit your taste. These range from ones that are very easy and quick to prepare to some that involve more time and skill. The choice is yours!

Can I drink alcohol on my two days?

There is absolutely no rule against this. However, it is not advisable as alcohol is high in calories and therefore likely to take too much of your allowance. And since it is recommended that we have at least two alcohol-free days per week, it makes sense to give your body an alcohol break.

What can I do if I suffer hunger-pangs on my low-calorie day?

Initially you may find this to be the case. This is easily avoided by drinking plenty of water or another calorie-free/low-calorie drink, hot or cold throughout the day, especially before a meal. Generally we should be drinking around eight glasses daily anyway but an extra intake will help on low calorie days. It doesn't have to be boring either: green tea is full of healthy antioxidants, calorie free and provides an excellent way of increasing water intake. And since our bodies depend on adequate water consumption, it is vital to drink sufficient. Another good way to deal with this is to have plenty of distractions like immersing yourself in a good book or turning to your favourite hobby.

After a short while your body will adjust to your new method of eating and hunger pangs should no longer be a significant problem.

What if I feel particularly hungry on the day after a lower-calorie day?

In the beginning that may be the case. However, listen carefully to your body and eat slowly. This way, you will undoubtedly find, as we did, that although you might think you can eat an enormous meal, you will not really be able to comfortably eat as much as you imagine. There is no need to over-compensate.

Can headaches be a problem when I'm eating less?

When you first start, with lower food intake on the low calorie days, you may experience the odd headache. However, frequent fluid intake will help to stave off headaches as well as avoiding possible constipation and fatigue.

Should I exercise on my reduced-calorie days?

Although exercise is very important, any strenuous exercise is best reserved for your five days of normal eating. However, there is evidence that people who do *some* form of exercise on their lower-calorie days burn more fat.

Chapter 2

Personally Speaking

Polly's Story

I had a very personal reason and interest for wanting to lose weight and maintain a healthy level, as obesity runs in my family, I feared becoming obese and dying prematurely as my mother sadly did. But I was sure there must be a way to get my weight down to an acceptable level *and to keep it there.*

I first heard about the 5:2 diet whilst watching an episode of Horizon, a UK science documentary television series. This particular programme was about dieting.

Munching on a packet of crisps washed down with a couple of glasses of wine, I was rapidly losing interest. The sight of a tired and strained Doctor Michael Mosley, the programme's presenter, sitting on a sunny Los Angeles beach whilst following a three-day, four-night fast, spoiled my enjoyment of my snack. He was not allowed to ingest anything other than lots of water, black tea and one 50 calorie cup-a-soup per day.

This was not a one-off fast; it would need to be repeated every couple of months to retain the beneficial results that a battery of health tests had revealed when he finished his fast.

I was just about to switch off when Dr Mosley announced rather downheartedly that using this method to lose weight and become healthier was not a long-term option he was prepared to undertake. He was determined to see whether any other, hopefully less stringent, route could maintain the same healthier results he'd achieved with his drastic fast.

He did indeed find a more palatable way that did not resort to prolonged fasting. At the Institute for Aging in Baltimore, Maryland, he was taken to see some mice that had been reared on 'feast and fast' days – or 'intermittent energy restriction days' as they were also termed. They were living much longer, showed far less risk of the early onset of brain disease than the control group and demonstrated much better memory recall in tests.

The researchers concluded that hunger really does make the brain sharper; and when questioned about the possibility of comparable results in humans following a similar regime, they said that the chances are very good to excellent of slowing down the aging process and giving many more years of healthy living.

In the interests of science and his own wellbeing, Dr Mosley practised the 5:2 diet over a five-week period.

The positive improvements were dramatic. Tests showed that his blood-sugar and cholesterol levels were now normal, whereas before he was bordering diabetic and might soon have to start medication to control his cholesterol level. His level of IGF-1, an insulin-related hormone, had reduced by fifty percent, greatly lowering his risk of cancers and diminishing the risk of dementia. These were life-changing results and Dr Mosley expressed his intention to continue eating this way.

I was sufficiently impressed that by the end of the programme I had already formed my intention to begin the 5:2 diet. Whatever diet I've previously tried has lasted at most a week before I've reverted to attempts to generally eat better, sticking to healthier cooking oils and bread spreads and eating lots of fruit and vegetables. But still, those stubborn extra pounds I had accumulated over the years refused to drop off – and worse, I felt guilty every time I ate a bar of chocolate, a cream cake or even the biscuit crumbs at the bottom of the tin.

The idea of restricting my calorie intake on just a couple of days a week, in fact any two days of my choice, and having more or less what I fancied on the other five, had, and still has, immense appeal.

I must admit I was rather sceptical about eating *anything* I wanted on my unrestricted-calorie days. So, although allowing myself ice-cream, baguettes and chocolate biscuits, I resolved to avoid the usual guilty feelings, when consuming my favourite foods, by including a good balance of fruit and vegetables, more portions of fish and poultry than red meat and going for a brisk walk or visiting the gym more often.

The day after making my decision, wasting no time I plunged into a 'fast' day. I ate no breakfast, had an apple for lunch and so saved most of my calories for my evening meal. With a raging headache and gnawing hunger pains, due to insufficient water intake, I spent most of the evening trying to figure out the correct number of calories per hundred grams for foods I had in stock, desperate to make a nutritious meal. By 9.30pm, when I had finally cobbled together a mixed salad and fish, I was utterly exhausted and confused about how many calories I had actually consumed that day.

Hours spent researching calorific values on various websites of a particular food item showed quite wide variations. And how was I supposed to know how they arrived at the number of calories for a 'piece' of fish, for example, when the weight was not specified?

My disorganised approach continued for the next couple of 'fast' days. On day two, having eaten what I thought was a small breakfast, a medium-sized lunch and drunk a few cups of tea with semi-skimmed milk, I totted up the calories and found that I'd used up my allotted 500 and had none left for the rest of the day. My husband did not fail to notice how bad-tempered I became while starving my body for the remainder of that day.

On the third day I got to the point where I had one calorie left for the day, which, in my intense desire to be mathematically accurate in my calorie consumption for the day, I was determined to use up. So I decided to eat one very small leaf of a Cos lettuce. I kidded myself that its laudanum content would help me sleep better. Later, however, I had a reality check and realised that it would actually take at least a kilo of lettuce to make a significant impact!

Day four was equally, though differently, disastrous. I won't bore you with the details. Suffice it to say that I grossly exceeded my intended calorie intake.

I finally took stock, scheduled Monday and Thursday for my two 'fast' days the following week and set about planning a structured, commonsense approach, one that would make life easy and not involve panicking or obsessing on my two low-calorie days. And instead of weighing myself on a daily basis I decided to limit myself to once a week. I resolved to integrate enjoyment and fun into the journey to becoming a healthier me.

I also realised that I would need to target my plan to match the goals of the mnemonic SMART – i.e. it would have to be

Specific

Measurable

Attainable

Relevant

Time-limited

This last goal triggered in me a sense of urgency, excitement and revived my waning enthusiasm.

After what was clearly a very confusing start to my attempt to embrace the 5:2 diet, which almost culminated in me consigning it to history, along with the other diets I've tried, I sat down and worked out a different approach: a SMART plan.

I no longer wanted to devote a large chunk of each day to working out afresh the calorific content of everything I ate or drank. I decided instead to invest time in devising a counter, which would ultimately simplify the entire process; it can be found at the end of this book, together with an alphabetical chart. The groundwork would then be done as far as calorie-counting was concerned and I could mix and match according to my tastes and calorie requirements.

One area of confusion occurred when I tried to find out why the packaging on many foods refers to calories as 'kcal'. The k is short for kilo, which means a thousand. A thousand calories. Does this mean that my innocent 20 calorie Ryvita crispbread slice actually contains 20,000 calories. Surely not. I looked the whole thing up on Wikipedia and discovered the scientific facts, which made my eyes glaze over a bit. All I need to report here is that for all practical, weight-watching purposes, 'kcal' and 'cal' mean the same thing as far as we are concerned, even if to a scientist they are different. So if you read on a packet that a meal contains 300kcal, that's 300 calories to you and me.

Over the course of twelve weeks, I did my research on grams and calories and devised meals for the twenty-four reduced calorie days in that period with as much variation of diet as possible and as little preparation as I could get away with. This also avoided the need to linger in the kitchen with the possible temptation of helping myself to 'snacks' from the cupboards. The keynote had to be simplicity as I got to grips with the 5:2 diet. I reckoned that after twelve weeks I could begin the cycle again.

When I began the 5:2 diet I left almost all my calorie intake until the evening. I found that my mood became affected and my blood sugar dropped owing to hunger, leaving me feeling quite faint. So I tried to spread food intake somewhat more evenly over the day. Plus I decided to have my evening meal reasonably early and avoid getting to bed late. The result was a far less hungry and happier me.

I also found that a glass of water, especially just before a meal, often relieved the urge to eat too much as it dampened down my hunger response. I drink on average two litres per day throughout the week, even on non-diet days.

I initially thought that after a reduced calorie day I would inevitably consume ten times the usual amount of food on my non-restricted days. My personal experience has shown this not to be the case. Before beginning the 5:2 diet, I wasn't really considering whether I actually wanted and/or appreciated everything I consumed in a day. It was only when I paid attention to what I ate and drank that my body had a chance to let me know that I'd had enough. Previously, I just used to plough on without listening to my body, stuffing in anything and everything, so to speak.

Another enormous plus of my new way of life was that I became increasingly aware of the taste of each morsel of food. I also began to savour the smell, texture and colour of everything I ingested.

At the start of each week I plan my two reduced calorie days, spacing them out to suit myself so that, for example, if I've been invited out for a meal, that day will not be one of them.

I have found that it is best to have my once-weekly weigh-in first thing in the morning before getting dressed. And if, occasionally, I gain slightly more weight (like when I went on holiday and had a week of no low-calorie days) I don't stress about it as I know the pounds will drop off again as soon as I return to keeping to my two reduced calorie days each week.

My energy levels have increased and I really appreciate my 'normal' days, making sure to include the odd pastry, bar of chocolate and glass of wine without any of the guilt I once felt about such 'treats' and knowing from experience that they do not interfere with my weight-loss program. As an extra bonus, I don't have to try to work out how to fit in the two recommended alcohol-free days each week. I know my glass of wine is high in calories so I don't include it in my two diet days in the week. This way I can appreciate it so much more when I do have a tipple!

I have now been a devotee of the 5:2 diet for over a year – far outstripping the length of time and sense of failure spent trying to follow a vast variety of other weight loss regimes over the years.

That is not to say, however, that it's been plain sailing all the time to date. Constipation and headaches were initially a problem which I quickly solved by drinking lots of water, fruit infusions and calorie-free green tea. Before I started the 5:2, green tea wasn't a beverage I would have rated but now I must confess to an addiction to it! Hot drinks also helped greatly at times when, during winter, I felt particularly cold. Calories produce heat, so it's understandable that I might sometimes feel somewhat colder on calorie-restricted days.

Having my meals at regular intervals on a low calorie day and generally reserving a reasonable number of calories for my evening meal overcame the bouts of irritability and anxiety that I noticed creeping in when I tried skipping lunch or sometimes not bothering to have any food at all until evening.

Initially, I became pre-occupied with thoughts of food, especially when I felt a strong pang of hunger (this disappeared after a few weeks when I began to settle into the diet) or watched someone tucking into a tasty dessert. But I reminded myself that I too could have this the next day and I turned my mind to an activity which did not involve food, such as writing, reading or creating colourful pictures.

In the beginning, I would wake up after a diet day and get myself a massive breakfast with the idea that, having eaten a lot less the previous day, I must need loads to fill me up. When I tried to get through the mound of cereal, toast and eggs I had prepared, I felt bloated and uncomfortable. I soon concluded that the amount of food I *thought* was necessary was utterly disproportionate to what I could *actually* manage. With time my stomach had begun to shrink and could not hold so much.

As I explored ways to maximise the use of my calorie allowance, I was delighted to come across almond milk, a beverage manufactured from ground almonds. It is an excellent substitute for dairy milk and massively lower in calories – especially the unsweetened variety. Using this frees up extra calories to add a bit more substance to a meal.

Tiredness became a problem too, at times. So I stopped pushing myself to exercise on reduced calorie days and began taking space for some 'me' time – not easy when so many things need doing. I invariably find though, that I get far more done on a day where I am conscious of doing only one thing - such as eating - at any given moment and giving it my entire attention for the duration.

Like so many others who have been on this diet for a while, I am considerably slimmer, having lost a total of 18 kilos (40 pounds). There have been some fluctuations but I've reached and am staying (within a whisker) at my target weight of 56 kilos (124 pounds).

I definitely have considerably more energy than I used to have and feel lighter and more contented. Whenever I see a photograph of myself taken a year or two ago, it reminds me of how much I have achieved with minimal effort.

I have considerably greater zest for life than before and look forward to each day of the healthier, happier, more productive life I'm leading. I wish you the same result!

Lucy's Story

Until my early thirties I didn't have a weight problem. In fact, I thought I was one of those lucky people who can eat whatever they like and still keep their weight at a steady, healthy level. So it never occurred to me to go on a diet. I just didn't need to.

Six pregnancies later, neglecting to follow all the sensible advice about post natal exercises and ignoring my monthly gym membership (although every month began with a resolution to work out regularly), my lack of attention to my body was obvious to all, especially me. Every visible part of me had travelled south and my five foot two inch frame had ballooned to an unhealthy twelve and a half stone. That's more than three stone over my ideal weight!

I began the long, uncomfortable journey of yoyo dieting. Any and every new diet regime I came across was, initially, to be my route to an even sleeker, slimmer healthier body than I'd had in the first place. I started each one with religious zeal and determination to succeed, convincing myself each time that this was it. I'd found the only diet that worked and suited my lifestyle at the same time.

And so it began. I worked my way rapidly through them one by one. I won't bore you with the entire list but among them featured:

the Hay, Acai Berry, the South Beach, Slim Fast, Gorgeously Green and the Lemon diets which were all-consuming for a week or two before I drifted back to my old well-trodden, familiar eating habits. And so the scales went up and down on a regular basis until I finally gave up. I concluded that I was one of many whose will power was strong initially but short-lived. Not only was I back to square one each time but I felt increasingly disheartened and began to worry a lot about my health.

I have now discovered that I am genetically pre-disposed to piling on the pounds, which is not to say that it's inevitable and that there is nothing I can do about it. I need to take responsibility for myself and cannot use that as an excuse. However, I do envy my husband who can eat whatever he fancies and who, just like all the relatives on his father's side, never puts on a dangerously unhealthy amount of weight. His father, uncles, aunts and grandparents all lived, or are living, long and productive lives. They all had (or have) a brilliant sense of humour too, though whether or not there is any significance in that I don't know!

My mother was morbidly obese and all my aunts were way overweight. Unfortunately, the heaviness of the problem extended beyond their size leading to serious health problems like diabetes and heart disease.

If I wanted to see my children develop their careers and enjoy any future grandchildren and great-grandchildren, it was crystal clear that I had to pull my socks up (if I could reach them), find a way to lose weight and hopefully live a long, active healthy life.

It was at this crucial point that the 5:2 diet hit the scene in a big way. Polly first told me about the diet, having already been on it for two months. She was so enthusiastic about it and said it was really working for her. To be honest it sounded too good to be true but the only way I could possibly find out if this were the case would be to give it a proper go myself.

And so I began with earnest zeal, whilst my family waited patiently for yet another diet to bite the dust.

The first couple of weeks were quite difficult. I was just eating a couple of scrambled eggs with a piece of ham for breakfast and having grilled chicken or fish and vegetables for dinner. I missed out lunch, had headaches, felt very tired and hungry and lacked energy. And I was on the point of giving up yet again.

But I decided, after listening to how Polly had coped in the early days, that it was now or never time and that I would think carefully before abandoning this diet. There was far too much at steak - sorry, stake...

My husband was adamant that he was not going on any diet with me so I had to try to make tasty meals for one. However, as I enjoy cooking, this became an interesting project, not just a time-consuming one. I spent hours researching the calorie content of ingredients for the recipes I was compiling and found that I was actually beginning to enjoy the process. I had never felt the slightest edge of happiness on any other diet.

I prepared in other ways ahead of my low calorie days - I had already decided to leave at least two days between them. I resolved to increase my water intake significantly. I began to compile a list of calorie free drinks and beverages low in calories so that I could give myself more options than just water for the two days. And, since the two low calorie days can be scheduled to suit yourself, I settled on Mondays and Fridays as best for me. If I were to be invited to a wedding or a party, or should my husband decide we need a night out, then I could always shift the days around.

So by week three I had the beginnings of a plan and felt considerably more in control. I had a few recipes for my low calorie days which kept me busy and able to cope with brief feelings of hunger whilst looking forward to the meal I was preparing. When I told my daughter-in-law about some of the recipes she asked for copies. I was delighted when she rang me and said that she had prepared one of the lunches the night before and enjoyed it at work the following day. She was looking forward to doubling the quantities of a dinner recipe and cooking it in the evening for the two of them.

And that is how my recipes in this book evolved over the ensuing weeks and months.

I discovered that apart from water, there were a lot of other drinks that added few or even no calories: black tea, green tea, fruit infusions, beef extract, yeast extract...

I have now been practising the 5:2 diet religiously for nine months, a feat I never thought possible. And I have joined the growing ranks of its fans. I have no more will power than I had before I started it but this time around I don't need to make a superhuman effort. It is a far easier diet than any I have ever attempted. I have lost weight steadily and feel so much lighter, in spirit as well as in body. It is like I've finally stopped constantly carrying around a small child (roughly the same weight as I shed). To put that in another context, try lifting forty-nine pounds of shopping and then imagine that weight distributed around your body permanently!

A couple of months ago I dropped to one low calorie day per week and I have found that the weight has not only stayed off but that my new healthy level remains fairly constant.

I have loads more energy, my mood has improved (ask my husband!), and I feel massively more motivated in so many ways. I am now able to exercise on a regular basis and join in more social activities than I have in ages.

On my five 'normal' days I try to follow a healthy Mediterranean eating style with plenty of fruit, vegetables and the odd glass or two of red wine. I continue to enjoy an occasional slice of tasty cake and a small piece of dark chocolate now and then. I never feel deprived or guilty since I know that the 5:2 diet allows for any choice I may make (within reason, of course).

The biggest surprise for me has been the fact that on my 'normal' days I am far less hungry than I used to be and have a considerably lower craving for sweet things.

I intend to continue this transformation of my eating habits for the foreseeable future. And, as if I needed any more evidence than I already have, my latest battery of blood tests results is the icing on the cake. I was taking a daily statin pill for twelve years because my cholesterol level was so high. I decided on a statin holiday three months ago, with my GP's approval, knowing that a few weeks off a statin for someone with no pre-existing heart disease was not a problem. Now my doctor has taken me off them since I have a level well within the normal range. He has also confirmed that my blood glucose is normal and that I no longer run the risk of diabetes.

When Polly introduced me to the concept of mindful eating I was quite excited about it. Putting it into practice has greatly enriched my experience of eating in general and preparing and eating food on my lower calorie days in particular. I'm now trying to apply its principles to every area of my life.

I sincerely hope (and expect) that like me you will feel lighter, fitter and more contented following the 5:2 diet in a mindful way.

Emily's Story

As a child I was teased mercilessly in the playground about my size. I wasn't exactly fat, just 'podgy' but the unkind remarks hurt. As a teenager I became increasingly conscious of my weight, especially as my brother and sister were both much slimmer than me. My self-esteem plummeted even lower and I developed a very poor body image.

As an adult I was lucky to marry someone who loved me for myself (and still does). However, because of my low self-esteem I became depressed and turned to eating for comfort. I soon billowed out and by the time I was thirty-five I weighed an unhealthy eighteen stone, completely unacceptable for my height of five foot six.

I tried every diet I came across but found it impossible to stick with any of them for very long, despite my determination. My weakness for my favourite foods, especially anything sweet, led to failure each time.

When Polly and Lucy first told me about the 5:2 diet, the idea sounded just too simple to work, even though they had both obviously lost weight. Surely something so straightforward would have been brought to light long before now were it truly effective, instead of all those complicated nutrient-specific regimes I'd been hopelessly working my way through for longer than I cared to remember? Indeed, had it not been for the endorsements by some recognised members of the scientific community, I may not even have attempted it – I'd had enough experience of failure.

However, I'm glad I went ahead with it! Not only did I find the 5:2 diet particularly easy to stick to, it also very quickly proved to be exceptionally effective. I lost weight surprisingly fast and found that I actually began to enjoy this new way of eating. I was spurred on even more by the fact that in the first couple of months I lost twenty-four pounds.

I think this is the easiest diet to follow, both in concept and in practice. And judging by its increasing popularity, I'm not the only one of this opinion!

As there is a certain amount of self-discipline required for the two low calorie days each week, I decided fairly early on to spice these days up by adding as much variety to what I ate and drank as possible. Obviously, the 500 calorie limit does cancel out certain high-calorie foods on your diet days; however, with a bit of creativity and variety these two days can become just as, if not even more, enjoyable.

One of the most effective ways I found to add this variety was by experimenting with different types of smoothies. They are a great way of packing healthy nutrients into a tasty drink, and can also be surprisingly filling. They are perfect for any meal, whether it be to give you the boost you need in the morning, to keep you going throughout the day or to help you relax in the evening.

Having always previously thought of smoothies as fruit-based drinks, I was pleasantly surprised to discover that actually there are many other foods that work just as well. In fact, something that became apparent very quickly was that often it was the really unexpected combinations that ended up with the most delicious drinks, as you will find in some of my recipes.

Like Polly and Lucy, I have managed to lose weight. After six months I'm halfway towards my target weight of 140 pounds, having lost 56 pounds. And the biggest spinoff has been that my self-esteem has improved immensely. I get up every day feeling better about myself than I ever did. My husband is delighted with my new-found confidence (which is just as well as he's footing the bill for new clothes to fit my slimmer frame!).

Listening to Polly and Lucy discussing mindful eating made me decide to try it for myself. I was surprised to find how much more enjoyable it made my experience of preparing and eating food.

Being kind to myself if I am having a bad day, which might be completely unrelated to food, is an effective way to deal with any distress. In the past I often used food to comfort myself but then I discovered rather more healthy ways to make myself feel better. It might be a bit of retail therapy but more often it's something that costs nothing, like going into the garden or walking in the park, listening to the various sounds, feeling the sun warming my skin and looking at the beauty of nature around me. I don't try to push away any feelings inside me – I simply notice them and accept that they are there but am aware of the need to look outward as well.

I am so glad that I decided to start the 5:2 diet. Thank you so much Polly and Lucy, for all your encouragement along the way. It really helps to have support, especially in the early days.

Chapter 3

Polly on Mindful Eating

And now to look at just how we can make doing this diet especially enjoyable by developing a mindful approach to it.

We spend a lot of time 'sleepwalking' through our lives. All too often, we are trying to multi-task or doing stuff on 'automatic pilot', not giving our full attention to any one thing.

How many times have you driven some place and wondered how you actually got there? That's not to suggest that you are a bad driver, it's just that things we do habitually like cleaning our teeth, dressing or everyday household chores frequently get done with our thoughts going off in different directions. Rarely are we completely focussed on the task in hand.

Whilst getting showered in the morning I might be thinking about what I'm going to do later in the day, something I did yesterday or what to wear. That doesn't mean I don't wash properly. It does mean, though, that I am not completely aware of what I am doing.

There have also been too many times when I have visited the ladies' toilet (the rest room) in a restaurant and on exiting have mindlessly ended up in the staff kitchen or another toilet, simply because I didn't notice the route I came in by!

Thomas Edison, the inventor of the electric light bulb, once asked several of his long-term employees what they noticed every day walking along the path from the road to his factory. When they had finished telling him everything they had seen around them on that fine spring morning, he was astonished to find that not one of them had mentioned the beautiful flowering cherry tree to one side of the path.

We can get so used to *doing* things that we can actually miss out heavily on *experiencing* them.

If we are being mindful, we are paying attention to what is actually going on, we are fully aware and awake in this moment. And realistically that's all there is – the here and now.

By being present we begin to wake up to the sensation of really living instead of switching off and disappearing somewhere else with our minds. We aren't in the past or the future but *here*, where it's all happening!

That's all very well, you might be thinking, but I have so many things to get done and I can't possibly shut out all the thoughts filling my head up. But that's the point – don't even *try* to.

Pause right now to watch what is going on in your mind whilst you are reading this page. Thoughts will come and go even in this short space of time but that's fine - just notice them passing through like clouds, refrain from making any judgement about them or getting caught up in their content and steer your focus gently back to this experience.

I suggest you read the next bit and then try it out for yourself, closing your eyes if it makes it easier for you. It's a short exercise, lasting only a few minutes, which has helped me to be mindful and which will, I believe, be helpful to you.

First, be *aware* of, and just observe, what thoughts are in your mind - watch them; then explore and try to name what you are feeling emotionally (happy, worried, self-critical...) and whether you feel tension in any part of your body – jaw, shoulders, buttocks...

Now *redirect your focus* to your breath – following its journey from the moment it enters your nostrils, flows down your windpipe and expands your chest and abdomen, to its way out, noting any change in temperature as it exits your nose.

If any thoughts crop up while you are doing this, just briefly acknowledge them rather than dwell on them and then return to your breath.

Finally, *scan your entire body*, including your posture and facial expression, and then *breathe into any muscular tension* allowing it to soften as you breathe out.

That's it. How do you feel now? Any different from before you began?

I try to practice this exercise about three times a day. It invariably ends up with my feeling more relaxed, more grounded in the present and at ease with myself.

I also become conscious of how much I tend to tighten up physically, quite involuntarily, as well as my tendency to be hard on myself.

 For example, like Emily I have in the past told myself repeatedly that I was fat, putting myself down in a manner that would be extremely hurtful if I did it to others.

And remembering to be kind to yourself is important, perhaps especially so when you are trying to follow a diet.

Mindfulness is worth reading about in much greater detail as it is an important and extremely useful life skill. However, for the purpose of this book I have tried to explain it as simply as possible so that you grasp enough to apply it to your mealtimes.

There are a good number of 'Mindful Eating' courses in the UK, France and the USA which must mean there is a need to take a different view of the essential, habitual activity of food consumption.

I have certainly found that taking time to apply mindful practice to my meals has improved not merely my attitude to and appreciation of what I eat but has also enabled me to 'slow down' a little in other things I do, as opposed to tearing mindlessly through the day.

I began to realise that my body would tell me when it needed food and there was no need (or inclination) to overload it. This added to my sense of wellbeing and my motivation to continue.

Once I realised that I no longer *really* wanted the large amounts of food I'd been used to before I started the 5:2 diet, I ate less on my five days of unrestricted calories and therefore achieved an increased weight loss. And I didn't feel deprived.

Whenever I tackle any task mindfully I achieve so much more than if I rush through it with half an eye on whatever I have to do next.

So you could start your reduced calorie days with the breathing exercise and then set about preparing your first meal with awareness, being fully focused on what you are doing from the moment you select the ingredients for your meal, through preparing them with interest, to choosing the crockery and cutlery.

When everything is prepared, sit down at a table and eat *without* engaging in any other activities at the same time (reading the newspaper, watching TV, listening to the radio...).

Appreciate the juxtaposition and appearance of the combination of foods on your plate and the origin of the products. A different selection of colours can look really appealing and inviting.

Thinking about the source of the food on your plate, the rain, sun and the farmers who helped produce what is in front of you can also make you thankful for it.

Notice each piece of food you select as you eat it: its colour, size, shape and smell.

Pay attention to the texture and taste of it in your mouth and where on your tongue it tastes differently.

And chew it slowly.

A meal concentrated on in this manner can be surprisingly and pleasurably different from one that is hurried through or consumed whilst doing other things. Even a small amount can feel and taste good. And because you have slowed the process down it feels more filling and is excellent for your digestion.

When you approach your two reduced calorie days like this you will discover that they become infinitely more satisfying.

Chapter 4

Polly's 24 Individual Menu Plans

Introduction

As they stand, the twenty-four days' worth of menus I've devised are designed for a woman to follow. However, they are equally suitable for men, who have the advantage of being able to choose another 100 calories-worth of nutrition. If you are following the diet with a partner, I would suggest that the man chooses something that isn't going to make the woman envious – or else eats his 100-calories-worth of chocolate or biscuits in private! Even better, settle for an extra chicken drumstick or a selection of fruit. After all, there are still five other days in the week for treats...

If there are things in these menus that are not to your taste, the counter and chart at the end of the book will enable you to choose substitutes in a mix-and match fashion, bearing in mind the fact that this may well mean adjusting some of the other parts of a day's menu to take account of any changes in the calorific values for the day. To facilitate this, I've listed the calorific values for each ingredient, as well as for the meal as a whole.

On the two lower calorie days days, calorie counting is of course necessary; but I want to stress here that it's important to understand that there is no need to get obsessed with numbers – the spirit of the diet is far more important than its minute details. Calorie-counting in the frenetic way I did on my third day of the 5:2 diet, would consume your mind as well as your time and is psychologically unhealthy. So if you are over or under by a few calories, there is no guilt attached. Commonsense should prevail and remind us that whoever came up with the numbers of calories to be consumed each day was not laying down some unbreakable law. Metabolic rates, the rate at which our bodies burn up energy, vary from person to person according to many factors, so there is nothing magic about the number 500 (or 600 for men). Certainly, from the viewpoint of getting the diet to work, we should aim to get reasonably close to these target numbers or we'll stray off course and little by little the whole purpose of the diet will be lost. But don't allow obsession to take over, either! In fact, as you'll notice, the daily totals of calories do not always amount to exactly 500.

At the end of the first page of menus ('Day 1') I've mentioned the need to drink water at regular intervals. This could have been added to every page but I didn't want to labour the point. It's enough to emphasise that drinking water is not only good for your system in many well-documented ways, but also really does help to alleviate hunger and keeps at bay the headaches so often associated with lower food intake.

Like most British people I like my cup of tea. If you share this taste, the fact that tea has zero calories means that you can indulge yourself even on reduced calorie days, though if you want milk in it you will have to factor it into your menu and allow for the extra calories. I've listed tea with milk in a couple of menus but to give you some idea of low or zero calorie alternatives I've included a wide variety of them. I wouldn't want you to get the idea that I'm recommending that you drink a different flavoured tea or infusion (sometimes called 'fruit teas') for every meal – imagine the number of opened packets you'd have in your cupboard if you used all the teabags I've mentioned! If you find something you like, there's nothing wrong with sticking with it.

I intended to steer clear of using brand names; having no

connection or vested interests with any food company, I've no particular reason to favour one brand over another. However, occasionally I found it necessary to use such names to identify the type of product. Had I, for instance, mentioned 'beef extract' or 'whole wheat biscuits' it might have caused confusion, whereas the words 'Bovril' and 'Weetabix' are so well anchored in the public consciousness (at least in the UK) that their use clarifies the meaning instantly. But it should be borne in mind that alternative brands, including supermarkets' own, are equally acceptable and often cheaper. And as you'll see from the sample menus, I added in a couple of branded ready meals that I've tried for myself and enjoyed. Occasionally, if you're pressed for time, a low calorie ready meal is a viable choice.

When it comes to vegetarian options, it is almost impossible not to name brands, since their formulation is often unique to one company or another. So to mention 'vegetarian sausage' is not enough in itself as can be seen if you compare the calorific values of the Linda McCartney and Quorn varieties. This does not in any way imply, however, that any one brand is better than another, just different.

The sweet-toothed among you will look in vain in these menus for chocolate or puddings; after all, the joy of the 5:2 diet is that these luxuries are permitted for the other five days in the week. However, there are those for whom tea or coffee (or even cereal) taken without a sweetener is a step too far. For them the good news is that there is a natural sweetener, which is produced from the leaves of the stevia plant (a member of the sunflower family). It is *three times* as sweet as sugar, is rated as having zero calories and is readily available in the UK under the brand name of Truvia.

When cooking, it's good to know that grilling, steaming or boiling add no calories to food. However, frying is a different matter: you have to take into account the amount of oil or fat used. Here again, a product has been developed that eases the burden or calorie-counting. There is a range of sprays available in most supermarkets labelled '1-Cal'. One spraying of this is equal to one calorie of oil. I use the olive oil spray but sunflower oil is also available. It should be borne in mind, of course, that you may need up to eight sprays to fry your food, but that's still only eight calories. And as one tablespoon of regular olive oil weighs in at a hefty 120 calories, the benefit becomes immediately obvious.

As to weights and measures, I've tried to make it easy but even here it's necessary to bring in a note of caution: other than exact weights, a lot is open to interpretation. Sometimes a familiar term, meant to signify a measure, can be almost meaningless in reality. What exactly is a 'pat' of butter? The question is not just a matter of being picky about words – since a 'pat' is said to contain 35 calories, getting this wrong makes quite a substantial difference. After trawling the internet, I found that a 'pat' is defined as being one inch square by a third of an inch thick. Perhaps there's an opening for someone who wants to go into business as a patmaker, making it easier to measure out our butter accurately!

At this point I need to make the necessary disclaimer: whilst I have taken care to check all my figures relating to calorific values and to give information that is as accurate as possible, I do not guarantee that they are exact. Where manufacturers' figures are available, I have used them. Where my research has revealed a degree of disagreement on the calorific content of certain foods, I've steered a middle course, generally rounding up or down to the nearest five. For foodstuffs with a content of fewer than twenty calories I've aimed to be as accurate as possible.

I have tried to vary the colours on your plate and a few sprigs of parsley, weighing in at a mere five calories or some mint leaves, which are virtually zero rated, not only add an extra bit of nourishment but also a lovely splash of colour as a garnish.

Furthermore, current scientific research suggests that the various natural colours of foods indicate the type of nutrients they contain. So it would seem that the greater the range of colours we consume, the wider our intake of nutrients.

To remove the impression of a having too little on my plate I treated myself to a set of smallish but very attractive plates. A fairly full small plate has a far better psychological effect than a half-empty large one! And I reserve these plates for my reduced calorie days to make these meals feel special.

To make your life easier it will help if you have a few basic measuring implements to hand: such high-tech devices as a teaspoon, a tablespoon, a measuring jug and a set of scales capable of weighing grams or ounces.

Day 1

BREAKFAST
1 medium slice cooked ham (35 cal)
Scrambled egg made with:
    1 large egg (75 cal)
    Semi-skimmed milk 10ml ($^1/_3$ fl.oz) (5 cal)
    Half tsp butter (15 cal)
    Salt (0 cal)
    Black pepper (pinch) (0 cal)

Black tea with slice of lemon (1 cal)
Total calories 131

LUNCH
1 medium carrot (25 cal)
1 kiwi fruit (45 cal)
10 grapes (35 cal)

Glass of water (0 cal)
Total calories 105

DINNER
1 medium size (126g / 4½ oz) potato, baked (110 cal)
    Top with 28g (1 oz) Cheddar cheese, grated (110 cal)
    and 1 tsp onion, raw chopped (4 cal)
    Garnish with mint (0 cal)
4 radishes (5 cal)
1 large red tomato, quartered (35 cal)

Green tea (0 cal)
Total calories 264

TOTAL CALORIES FOR DAY: 500

Day 2

BREAKFAST
10g ($^1/_3$ oz) porridge oats (40 cal)
    60ml (2 fl.oz) soya milk (30 cal)
    Add blueberries 56g (2 oz) (25 cal)
    Stevia to sweeten (0 cal)
Microwave for 2 min (based on 700W). Add blueberries.
Microwave for further 30 sec & serve. Timings are approximate
and will vary according to the power of your microwave. For a
smoother consistency add a little water as desired.

Mug of green tea (0 cal)
Total calories 95

LUNCH
1 large egg, boiled (75 cal)
1 round medium-sliced wholemeal bread toasted (70 cal)
1 tsp olive spread (25 cal)

Cup of tea with semi-skimmed milk (15 cal)
Total calories 185

DINNER
1 chicken drumstick, cooked skinless (75 cal)
84g (3 oz) cauliflower (dry measure) steamed (50 cal)
1 medium carrot, steamed (25 cal)
84g (3 oz) peas, frozen, cooked (35 cal)
6 cherry tomatoes (20 cal)
4 slices cucumber (4 cal)

Bovril (beef extract), 1 tsp in mug of hot water, to drink (10 cal)
Total calories 219

TOTAL CALORIES FOR DAY: 499

Day 3

BREAKFAST
1 medium slice wholemeal toast (75 cal)
    Top with 112g (4 oz) canned chopped tomatoes, heated (25 cal)
    Garnish with fresh mint (0 cal)

Green tea (0 cal)
Total calories 100

LUNCH
3 low-fat cream crackers (55 cal)
    Top with 35g (1¼ oz) mini tub extra light Philadelphia soft cheese (38 cal)
84g grated carrot (25 cal)

Diet cola (0 cal)
Total calories 118

DINNER
Pasta Salad:
    56g (2 oz) penne pasta   (dry weight) (175 cal)
    56g (2 oz) peas, cooked from frozen (24 cal)
    1 tsp chopped parsley (1 cal)
    1 tsp chopped chives (1 cal)
    Juice of ½ lemon (10 cal)
    ½ tbsp olive oil (60 cal)
    1 tbsp onion, chopped (10 cal)
Cook pasta & peas. Drain & rinse, combine & mix with other ingredients. Cover & store in fridge until required. Serve cold.

Sparkling water (0 cal)
Total calories 281

TOTAL CALORIES FOR DAY: 499

Day 4

BREAKFAST
10g ($^1/_3$ oz) porridge oats (40 cal)
    60ml (2 fl.oz) soya milk (30 cal)
    84g (3 oz) strawberries (25 cal)
    Stevia to sweeten (0 cal)
Microwave for 2 min (based on 700W). Add strawberries.
Microwave for further 30 sec & serve. Timings are approximate
and will vary according to the power of your microwave. For a
smoother consistency add a little water as desired.

Lime & Ginger infusion (2 cal)
Total calories 97

LUNCH
1 large apple (110 cal)
1 kiwi fruit (45 cal)

Coffee, black filtered (1 cal)
Total calories 156

DINNER
84g (3oz) Atlantic salmon steak (140 cal)
    Drizzle with ¼ tsp olive oil (10 cal)
    Season with salt & black pepper (0 cal)
    & 1 crushed garlic clove (5 cal)
Bake in foil parcel for 25 min on medium high heat. Serve with:
100g (3½ oz) broccoli (35 cal)
100g (3½ oz) sliced carrot (cooked or raw) (35 cal)
6 slices cucumber (5 cal)
    Garnish with parsley (1 cal)

Tea with semi-skimmed milk (15 cal)
Total calories 246

TOTAL CALORIES FOR DAY: 499

Day 5

BREAKFAST
1 small egg, boiled (55 cal)
1 medium slice wholemeal toast (75 cal)
   Spread with 1 tsp peanut butter (30 cal)

Earl Grey tea (0 cal)
Total calories 160

LUNCH
Fresh fruit mixed salad:
   Small apple, 1 chopped (55 cal)
   Kiwi fruit, 1 peeled & sliced (45 cal)
   Strawberries, chopped, 84g (3 oz) (20 cal)
   Lemon juice 1 tsp (1 cal)

Diet cola (0 cal)
Total calories 121

DINNER
1 small lemon sole 84g (3 oz) grilled (80 cal)
   Garnish with parsley (1 cal)
   and 1 slice of lemon (1 cal)
   Season with salt, pepper (0 cal)
100g (3½ oz) broccoli steamed (35 cal)
100g (3½ oz) carrot steamed (35 cal)
90g ((3¼ oz) baby new potatoes (65 cal)

Cucumber, Nettle & Aloe Vera infusion (2 cal)
Total calories 219

TOTAL CALORIES FOR DAY: 500

Day 6

BREAKFAST
10g ($^1/_3$ oz) porridge oats (40 cal)
    60ml (2 fl.oz) semi skimmed milk (30 cal)
    84g (3 oz) of fresh raspberries (30 cal)
    Stevia to taste (0 cal)
Microwave for 2 min sec (700W). Add raspberries. Microwave for further 30 sec & serve. Timings are approximate. For a smoother consistency add a little water as desired.

Black coffee, instant (2 cal)
Total calories 102

LUNCH
Hardboiled egg, large, sliced (75 cal)
Iceberg lettuce, 84g (3 oz), shredded (5 cal)
2 low-fat (1%) crackers (35 cal)
    Spread with 1 triangle extra-light processed cheese (20 cal)
3 cherry tomatoes (10 cal)
6 slices cucumber (5 cal)

Green tea (0 cal)
Total calories 150

DINNER
100g (3½ oz) lean sirloin steak, grilled (185 cal)
84g (3oz) mushrooms, grilled (12 cal)
227g (8 oz) canned chopped tomatoes (50 cal)

Sparkling water (0 cal)
Total calories 247

TOTAL CALORIES FOR DAY: 499

Day 7

BREAKFAST
Weetabix, 1 biscuit (65 cal)
    75ml (2½ fl.oz) almond milk (10 cal)
    Stevia to taste (0 cal)

Strawberry & mango infusion (2 cal)
Total calories 77

LUNCH
Leek & potato cup soup, low fat, 1 sachet (55 cal)
1 large plum (35 cal)

Sparkling water (0 cal)
Total calories 90

DINNER
100g (3½ oz) smoked haddock, baked (115 cal)
50g (1³/₄ oz) (dry weight) brown rice, long-grain (185 cal)
56g (2 oz) peas, cooked from frozen (24 cal)
3 spring onions (5 cal)
56g (2 oz) iceberg lettuce (3 cal)

Green tea (0 cal)
Total calories 332

TOTAL CALORIES FOR DAY: 499

Day 8

BREAKFAST
28g (1 oz) corn flakes (110 cal)
    75ml (2½ fl.oz) almond milk, unsweetened (10 cal)
    Stevia to taste (0 cal)

Tea with skimmed milk (10 cal)
Total calories 130

Mid morning: Filtered black coffee **1 cal**

LUNCH
Yoghurt, vanilla, fat-free, 125g (4½ oz) pot (65 cal)
1 small apple (55 cal)
1 stick celery (5 cal)

Diet cola (0 cal)
Total calories 125

DINNER
130g (4½ oz) skinless chicken breast, grilled (190 cal)
Asparagus, 4 spears, steamed (15 cal)
168g (6 oz) cauliflower, steamed (30 cal)
56g (2 oz) mushrooms, grilled (8 cal)
    Garnish with 1 tsp chives (1 cal)

Green tea (0 cal)
Total calories 244

TOTAL CALORIES FOR DAY: 500

Day 9

BREAKFAST
1 lean rasher back bacon, grilled (65 cal)
1 large egg, scrambled as Day 1 (95 cal)
Tomato, medium, halved & grilled (25 cal)

Coffee, black filtered (1 cal)
Total calories 186

LUNCH
3 sticks celery (15 cal)
   Top with 84g (3 oz) cottage cheese, low fat (68 cal)
2 small beet, cooked (30)
4 radishes (5 cal)

Black tea (0 cal)
Total calories 118

DINNER
Mixed salad:
   Hardboiled egg, large sliced (75 cal)
   56g (2 oz) grated carrot (25 cal)
   1 medium tomato, quartered (25)
   ½ red pepper, small sliced (10 cal)
   ½ yellow pepper, small sliced (10 cal)
   4 slices cucumber (4 cal)
   84g (3 oz) iceberg lettuce, shredded (5 cal)
Dressing:
   1 tsp olive oil (40 cal)
   1 tsp lemon juice (1 cal)

Blueberry & Apple fruit infusion (2 cal)
Total calories 197

TOTAL CALORIES FOR DAY: 501

Day 10

BREAKFAST
Banana smoothie:
    Yoghurt, plain, low fat 150g (5 oz) pot (80 cal)
    Banana, small (70 cal)
    ½ tsp honey (10 cal)
    30ml (1 fl.oz) almond milk (4 cal)
    Blend & serve

Black coffee, instant (2 cal)
Total calories 166

LUNCH
Spring vegetable cup soup, 1 sachet (45 cal)
1 stick celery (5 cal)

Sparkling water (0 cal)
Total calories 50

DINNER
Omelette:
    2 medium eggs (130 cal)
    1 small, diced onion (20 cal)
    ½ yellow pepper, small, chopped (10 cal)
    Salt & pepper to taste (0 cal)
    Pinch of dried mixed herbs (1 cal)
    28g (1 oz) grated cheddar cheese (110 cal)
    2 tbsp water (0 cal)
    1 cal olive oil spray, 4 sprays (4 cal)
    Garnish with watercress (1 cal)
Serve with 84g (3 oz) leaf lettuce (5 cal)

Blackcurrant & Mint infusion (2 cal)
Total calories 283

TOTAL CALORIES FOR DAY: 499

Day 11

BREAKFAST
70g (1½ oz) All-bran cereal (67 cal)
    75ml (2½ fl.oz) semi-skimmed milk (37 cal)
    Stevia to taste (0 cal)

Black tea (0 cal)
Total calories 104

LUNCH
2 Ryvita slices original crispbread (40 cal)
    1 pat butter or margarine (35 cal)
    Top with 5 slices cucumber (4 cal)

Diet cola (0 cal)
Total calories 79

DINNER
200g (7 oz) potato, baked with skin (190 cal)
    1 pat butter or margarine (35 cal)
    Topped with 56g (2oz) canned tuna (90 cal)
    and 1 spring onion, chopped (1 cal)
    Garnish with parsley (1 cal)

Rooibos Red tea (0 cal)
Total calories 317

TOTAL CALORIES FOR DAY: 500

Day 12

BREAKFAST
½ grapefruit, sprinkled with stevia (40 cal)
1 small egg, poached (55 cal)
1 medium slice white bread, toasted (55 cal)
    Low fat spread, 1 pat (35 cal)

Vanilla black tea (0 cal)
Total calories 185

LUNCH
10 grapes (35 cal)
28g (1 oz) strawberries (9 cal)
1 passion fruit (17cal)
1 small apple (55 cal)

Green tea with jasmine (0 cal)
Total calories 116

DINNER
2 fish fingers (110 cal)
56g (2 oz)fresh egg noodles, ready cooked (38 cal)
56g (2 oz) peas, cooked from frozen (24 cal)
84g (3 oz) cooked diced beetroot (25 cal)

Black tea lemon spiced (0 cal)
Total calories 197

TOTAL CALORIES FOR DAY: 498

Day 13

BREAKFAST
10g ($^1/_3$ oz) porridge oats (40 cal)
    60ml (2 fl.oz) semi skimmed milk (30 cal)
    14g (½ oz) raisins (46 cal)
Microwave for 2 min sec (700W). Add raisins. Microwave for further 30 sec & serve. Timings are approximate. For a smoother consistency add a little water as desired.

English breakfast tea (black) (0 cal)
Total calories 116

LUNCH
2 apricots (30 cal)
1 satsuma (20 cal)
1 large plum (35 cal)

Ceylon Orange Pekoe tea (0 cal)
Total calories 85

DINNER
2 Quorn vegetarian sausages, grilled (140 cal)
1 potato waffle, 56g (2 oz), grilled (95 cal)
Small onion, sliced (20 cal)
56g (2 oz) button mushrooms (8 cal)
    Sauté onion & mushrooms in 1-cal spray, 6 sprays (6 cal)
84g (3 oz) cauliflower, steamed (30 cal)
    Garnish with fresh parsley (1 cal)

Green tea with apple & pear (0 cal)
 Total calories 300

TOTAL CALORIES FOR DAY: 501

Day 14

BREAKFAST
Weetabix, 1 biscuit (65 cal)
    75ml (2½ fl.oz) almond milk (10 cal)
    Stevia to taste (0 cal)

Black tea (0 cal)
Total calories 75

LUNCH
1 small apple (55 cal)
1 stick celery (5 cal)
6 cherry tomatoes (20 cal)

Diet cola (0 cal)
Total calories 80

DINNER
Bisto Shepherd's Pie frozen ready meal (341 cal)
    Garnish with mint leaves (0 cal)

Camomile, Fennel & Liquorice infusion (2 cal)
Total calories 343

TOTAL CALORIES FOR DAY: 498

Day 15

BREAKFAST
28g (1oz) Grape Nut cereal (100 cal)
    75 ml (2½ fl.oz) skimmed milk (28 cal)
    Stevia to taste (0 cal)

Green tea (0 cal)
Total calories 125

LUNCH
2 slices Ryvita Original crispbread (40 cal)
    Top with 40g (1½ oz) low-fat cottage cheese (30 cal)
1 medium tomato (25 cal)

 Lipton Morocco Mint & Spice infusion (3 cal)
Total calories 98

DINNER
70g (2½ oz) lamb leg, lean roasted (135 cal)
84g (3 oz) new potatoes, boiled (63 cal)
84g (3 oz) peas, cooked from frozen (35 cal)
84g (3 oz) broccoli, steamed (45 cal)

Earl Grey Tea (0 cal)
Total calories 278

TOTAL CALORIES FOR DAY: 501

Day 16

BREAKFAST
28g (1oz) Rice Krispies (110 cal)
    75ml (2½ fl.oz) semi-skimmed milk (37 cal)
    Stevia to taste (0 cal)

Aniseed, Fennel & Liquorice infusion (2 cal)
Total calories 149

LUNCH
1 medium banana (105 cal)
2 apricots (30 cal)
1 medium plum (30cal)

Earl Grey tea (0 cal)
Total calories 165

DINNER
1 Linda McCartney Veg. Sausage (95 cal)
84g (3 oz) new potatoes, boiled (63 cal)
½ small red onion, sliced (10 cal)
    Fry onion in 4 sprays 1-cal oil (4 cal)
84g (3 oz) cabbage steamed (12 cal)

Black coffee, instant (2 cal)
Total calories 186

TOTAL CALORIES FOR DAY: 500

Day 17

BREAKFAST
28g (1oz) cornflakes (110 cal)
    75ml (2½ fl.oz) almond milk (10 cal)
    Stevia to taste (0 cal)

Green tea (0 cal)
Total calories 120

LUNCH
Ginger Smoothie:
    60ml (2 fl.oz) pineapple juice (34 cal)
    120ml (4 fl.oz) orange juice (60 cal))
    1 small banana, chopped (70 cal)
    ½ tsp grated root ginger (1 cal)
    Ice cubes (0 cal)
    Blend all ingredients thoroughly

Earl Grey tea, bergamot flavoured (0 cal)
Total calories 165

DINNER
1 pack Quorn Cottage Pie, chilled ready meal, 300g (213 cal)
    Garnish with parsley (1 cal)

Sparkling water (0 cal)
Total calories 214

TOTAL CALORIES FOR DAY: 499

Day 18

BREAKFAST
45g (1½ oz) muesli, Alpen Original (170 cal)
    75ml (2½ fl.oz) almond milk (10 cal)

Black tea (0 cal)
Total calories 180

LUNCH
12 grapes (42 cal)
1 small peach (35 cal)
1 tangerine (35 cal)

Sparkling water (0 cal)
Total calories 112

DINNER
84g (3oz) halibut, grilled/broiled, with butter (140 cal)
1 medium tomato, grilled (25 cal)
    Season with salt & pepper (0 cal)
    Garnish with parsley (1 cal)
3 sticks celery (15 cal)
4 radishes (5 cal)
1 yellow pepper, sliced (20 cal)
56g (2 oz) iceberg lettuce (3 cal)

Green tea, lemon flavoured (0 cal)
Total calories 209

TOTAL CALORIES FOR DAY: 501

Day 19

BREAKFAST
1 Shredded Wheat (75 cal)
    75ml (2½ fl.oz) almond milk (10 cal)
    Stevia to sweeten (0 cal)

Blackcurrant, Ginseng & Vanilla infusion (2 cal)
Total calories 87

LUNCH
3 sticks celery (15 cal)
with dip of 1 mini tub extra light Philadelphia soft cheese, 35g (38)
1 medium orange (60 cal)
1 medium Asian pear (50 cal)

Sparkling water (0 cal)
Total calories 163

DINNER
1 medium, cooked chicken drumstick, skinless, (75 cal)
84g (3 oz) peas cooked from frozen (35 cal)
1 medium corn on cob (100 cal)
    Top with 1 pat margarine (35 cal)

Black instant coffee (2 cal)
Total calories 247

TOTAL CALORIES FOR DAY: 497

Day 20

BREAKFAST
1 large boiled egg (75 cal)
1 slice crispbread, (20 cal)
   Spread with 1 tsp peanut butter (30 cal)

Strawberry & mango infusion (2 cal)
Total calories 127

LUNCH
Cup-a Soup, spring vegetable, 13g (½ oz) sachet (45 cal)
1 stick celery (5 cal)

Coffee, black filtered (1 cal)
Total calories 51

DINNER
84g (3 oz) lamb's liver (190 cal)
1 small onion, sliced (20 cal)
1 Cal Oil spray, 7 sprays (7 cal)
   Fry liver & onions together
84g (3 oz) potato, mashed with skimmed milk, (100 cal)
Mustard 1 tsp (5 cal)

Black tea (0 cal)
Total calories 322

TOTAL CALORIES FOR DAY: 500

Day 21

BREAKFAST
1 small egg (55 cal)
Fry in 1 cal olive oil spray, 2 sprays (2 cal)
1 slice wholemeal bread, toasted (70 cal)
Spread with 1 tsp olive spread (25 cal)

Black tea (0 cal)
Total calories 152

LUNCH
1 crumpet, toasted (90 cal)
Top with 1 tsp honey (20 cal)

Blueberry & Apple infusion (2 cal)
Total calories 112

DINNER
1 rollmop herring, as *starter* (90 cal)

1 medium (100g / 3½ oz) potato, baked with skin (110 cal)
Top with 1 tsp chives, chopped (1 cal)
28g (1 oz) mushrooms, grilled (4 cal)
1 medium carrot, grated (25 cal)
84g (3 oz) iceberg lettuce (5 cal)

Diet cola (0 cal)
Total calories 235

TOTAL CALORIES FOR DAY: 499

Day 22

BREAKFAST
10g ($^1/_3$ oz) porridge oats (40 cal)
  Soya milk 60ml (2 fl.oz) (30 cal)
  Stevia extract to sweeten (0 cal)
  70g (2½ oz) blackberries (30 cal)
Microwave for 1 min 30 sec. Add blackberries.
Microwave for further 30 sec & serve. Timings are approximate.
For a smoother consistency add a little water as desired.

Black instant coffee (2 cal)
Total calories 102

LUNCH
2 rice cakes (60 cal)
  Top with 1 triangle extra light processed cheese, (20 cal)

Sparkling water (0 cal)
Total calories 80

DINNER
112g (4 oz) turkey roast, cooked (170 cal)
112g (4 oz) new potatoes dry roasted (84)
1 medium carrot, steamed (25)
84g (3 oz) peas cooked from frozen (35 cal)

Green tea with slice of lemon (1 cal)
Total calories 315

TOTAL CALORIES FOR DAY: 497

Day 23

BREAKFAST

1 medium slice white bread, toasted (55 cal)
    Topped with 1 pat butter, low fat (35 cal)

Green tea (0 cal)
Total calories 90 cal

LUNCH
10 cherries (50 cal)
1 large plum (35 cal)
140g (5 oz) strawberries (45 cal)

Rooibos Tea (0 cal)
Total calories 130

DINNER
2 rashers back bacon, lean (130 cal), grilled
1 medium tomato, halved and grilled (25 cal)
28g (1 oz) mushrooms, grilled (4 cal)
1 small egg (55 cal)
    Fry in 1 cal oil, 2 sprays (2 cal)
84g (3 oz) new potatoes, boiled (63 cal)

Sparkling water (0 cal)
Total calories 279

TOTAL CALORIES FOR DAY: 499

Day 24

BREAKFAST
1 slice medium white bread, toasted (55 cal)
   Top with 112g (4 oz) chopped tomatoes, heated (25 cal)

Options low fat chocolate drink (40 cal)
Total calories 121

LUNCH
1 medium Asian pear (50 cal)
1 small apple (55 cal)
100g (3½ oz) honeydew melon (30 cal)
1 small peach (35 cal)

Sparkling water (0 cal)
Total calories 170

DINNER
Sweet Pepper,Tomato & Onion Omelette:
   2 small eggs (110 cal)
   1 tsp diced onion (4 cal)
   ½ yellow pepper, chopped (10 cal)
   ½ red pepper, chopped (10 cal)
   ½ green pepper, chopped (10 cal)
   6 cherry tomatoes, halved (20 cal)
   1 tsp olive/vegetable oil (40 cal)
   Salt & pepper (0 cal)
   Garnish with parsley (1 cal)
   an*d* 1 tsp chives,,chopped (1 cal)
Sauté peppers, tomatoes & onions lightly in oil, then pour on beaten eggs. Cook, garnish & serve

Camomile & Spear mint infusion (2 cal)
Total calories 208

TOTAL CALORIES FOR DAY: 499

Chapter 5

Lucy's Tasty Recipes For One

The purpose of this chapter is to provide a range of enjoyable, tasty, calorie-controlled recipes for one person.

When I started to follow the 5:2 diet I spent a lot of time seeking out recipes that I could use myself. This was harder than you might imagine. Often I would encounter a dish that sounded delicious, only to read that it fed eight to ten people. Dividing ingredients by ten was not always practical – making a casserole for one person, for instance, is not easy unless you make more than you want and store or freeze the rest.

So I spent some time experimenting and adapting to find out what worked and tasted good for my meal and what didn't.

A couple of recipes make more than you will need at the time: the banana muffins, for instance. But in these cases the extra portions are ones that store easily – or that your nearest and dearest will eat even before they get that far. And doubling the amounts is easily done if you want to share a meal with someone else.

Of course, your entire calorie allowance can be used up in one meal or two. But I found that a three-meals-a-day regime suits me best, as I guess it will for many other people, and that is how I have set out the meals in this section.

Each calorie-restricted day has as a complete menu of three meals. The calorie value for each meal is given, as is the total for the whole day.

You will notice that the daily total does not always equal 500 calories exactly. Don't get obsessive about a couple of calories here or there. One calorie by itself is of little significance. As long as you reach a total very close to your target (500 calories for a woman, 600 for a man) you are on course to lose weight and gain from all the other benefits of the 5:2 diet.

It would be virtually impossible to write a set of daily menus to suit everyone and I recognise that some of the menus may contain a meal that may not be to your taste. So in the reference section at the end of the book I have listed all the breakfasts, lunches and dinners separately, together with the calorie count of each one given in brackets. That should enable you to mix and match as you wish – simply make sure that your chosen meals for the day add up to no more than your allotted calorie allowance.

Almost all the ingredients listed are easily available – I've tried to steer clear of anything that might prove problematic to source. An ingredient that a few people may occasionally find difficult to obtain in the UK is the Edamame beans. I know, however, that Waitrose and many health-food shops stock them. In the USA they are being hailed as a super-food (as blueberries are).

Not so long ago, the sweet-toothed dieter was left with a rather unappealing choice: no sugar at all or artificial sweeteners. Mercifully, this is no longer the case. There are several natural sweeteners available that are low in calorific value and one that is completely calorie free, called stevia. This may sound like a trendy name for a baby girl but in fact it is an extract from the leaves of a plant of that name, which grows in North and South America. In the UK it is marketed under a number of brand names the easiest to find being Truvia, as Polly mentioned earlier. In the US the main brand appears to be Sweet Leaf. Having used stevia extract myself I can say that it tastes good and is completely free from the artificial overtones that characterise many other sweeteners. It is extremely sweet though, and should be used sparingly – a third of a teaspoon is equivalent to a full teaspoon of sugar!

As Polly has also mentioned, the use of 1-cal oil sprays can cut down your calorie consumption considerably.

If your day's total on any day is below 500 (men read 600), you have the leeway to enjoy drinks with some calorie count. Filtered coffee taken black contains only 1 calorie, but add a splash of semi-skimmed milk and it rises to about 15. Using skimmed milk takes this down to 10 calories. These need to be factored into your day's total. To help you with drinks you might enjoy on a calorie-restricted day, I have compiled a list. It's worth noting that even within the zero-calorie list there is a reasonable choice.

Zero Calorie Drinks:

Still water, tap or bottled

Sparkling mineral water

Black tea

Earl Grey tea

Rooibos (Red Bush) tea

Green tea

Diet cola

Diet soda

Iced tea, black

There is a range of zero-rated flavoured canned drinks marketed under the brand name Zevia. Their website lists fifteen flavours. They apparently contain natural flavourings and no artificial sweeteners, using instead the previously-mentioned stevia extract. They are manufactured in the United States and have now made their first appearance in the UK online at Ocado. I am not endorsing them here, simply showing the wide range of options available for zero-calorie drinks.

Drinks containing calories:

Flavoured green tea (1)

Fruit infusions (fruit teas) (2-4)

Coffee, filtered, black (1)

Coffee, instant, black (2)

Low calorie fruit squashes (below 10)

Tea with skimmed milk (10)

Yeast extract (e.g. Vegex, Marmite, Vegemite), 1 tsp (10)

Tea with semi-skimmed milk (15)

And, if your day's calories allow, there are instant 40-calorie hot chocolate drinks available. You just add hot water.

Although this list looks quite short, a few minutes spent at the tea section of your local supermarket/grocery store will reveal a vast range of flavoured infusions which should satisfy almost all tastes – strawberry, camomile, fennel, peppermint, peach, ginger... the list goes on and on. None of them contains more than 4 calories and placing a mint leaf or two on top will enhance the flavour as well as the appearance and give it that 'special' feel. And don't forget stevia if you prefer your drinks sweet!

As we've already mentioned, drinking plenty of water is essential to keep us healthy. Every organ in the body needs it. The skin is not only the largest organ, it's also the only visible one and good hydration keeps it looking and feeling good. Drinking lots of water is also an important factor in enabling the body to eliminate harmful toxins.

What of the extra hundred a man is allowed each calorie-restricted day? Well, when I tell you that one glass of fresh orange juice or one banana can account for the whole hundred it doesn't seem that much, does it? He can, of course, opt instead for a couple of squares of chocolate, a chicken drumstick, a small piece of cheese or maybe an apple and tangerine. And since vegetables are generally pretty low in the calorie stakes, a large extra portion of mixed veg may well help to keep his tummy satisfied.

Many of the recipes list salt and pepper as ingredients. This should not be taken as meaning that I think salt is so great that I want you to take in lots of the stuff. Doctors are regularly warning us of the danger to our blood pressure (and therefore our continued wellbeing) of over-consumption of salt and generally I use it very sparingly, if at all. However, it's listed, along with its sidekick pepper, as a seasoning agent to enhance the flavour of food and not to swamp it. In other words, please use salt with due caution.

It is also worth mentioning here that some of the recipes use vegetable or chicken stock. If you are one of those cooks who make their own stock, that's great. However, many of us will reach for the ready-made commercial varieties that come in the form of cubes or gel. If that is so in your case, please take a moment to read on the packaging the recommended dilution with water, since the first ingredient listed in these products is salt – which means that salt is the most plentiful ingredient. Surprisingly, even the low salt variety still lists salt as the main ingredient. So please don't be tempted to use less water simply because the recipe doesn't use that much.

I haven't included in any of the instructions the need to wash fruit and vegetables because I'm assuming you'll do that anyway!.

To make your restricted calorie day easier to manage, be sure to look at its menu for a day or two ahead so that if a meal involves any shopping or preparation the day before (for instance, if you are wanting a lunch to take to work) you are well prepared with everything you require. You can't make toast without bread!

Where microwave cookers are mentioned, the timings are based on a 750 watt device and if yours differs from this, cooking times will need to be adjusted accordingly. All timings for *any* cooking, whether frying, baking, grilling/broiling, boiling or microwaving, are of course approximate. There's no purpose to be served watching a meal turn black and charred just to observe the stated times. Appliances vary as does almost everything else in life!

I'm assuming that the reader will already have all the usual cooking utensils. But there are some recipes that require other devices such as a blender. It will come in handy for Emily's smoothies, too. Emily gives advice in her chapter on choosing a suitable blender. And to make juicing fruit and the occasional vegetable easier I'm also going to suggest a juice extractor, even though it's possible to pulp most things in a blender and sieve them to get the juice you want (which is a messy way of doing it!). A ridged griddle pan, a wok and mortar and pestle are also useful additions to your collection. And don't forget an accurate set of scales: electronic ones can be bought quite cheaply and are indispensible for weighing small quantities.

It will also help to have some potted herbs on the kitchen windowsill, including mint, coriander, parsley and basil, from which you can freely pick the leaves.

Choosing your favourite crockery and glassware, as well as your finest cutlery, and mindfully taking care with presentation, will enhance the experience of your reduced-calorie days.

I've arranged the layout of recipes so that you don't have to turn pages in the middle of one during your cooking sessions.

So that's it – now it's over to you to enjoy the recipes that follow and to lose weight and gain in health as you do.

Bon Appétit!

Menu 1

Breakfast - 100 calories

Grapefruit and Pistachio Delight

1 medium grapefruit
10g (about ½ teaspoon) chopped pistachio nuts
Stevia to taste

- Peel the grapefruit and divide into segments
- Sprinkle with pistachios
- Add Stevia to taste

Lunch - 120 calories

Cucumber, Orange and Mint Smoothie

1 small apple
½ cucumber
2 small oranges
Mint leaves to taste
Ice cubes (optional)

- Slice the apple and cucumber into thick chunks
- Extract the juice using a juicer
- Squeeze the oranges
- Put all the juice in a blender together with the mint leaves and whisk at high speed for a few seconds
- Add ice cubes to chill

Dinner - 279 calories

Tangy Tomato and Mozzarella Salad

5 cherry tomatoes, halved
2 spring onions, trimmed and chopped
½ tablespoon vinegar (preferably balsamic)
15 ml (3 teaspoons) extra virgin olive oil
56g (2oz) mozzarella cheese, cubed
5 sprigs parsley, curly or flat
Several leaves fresh basil
Salt
Ground black pepper

- Put the tomato halves and the spring onions into a large bowl
- Sprinkle the vinegar and oil over the contents of the bowl and toss thoroughly
- Add the cubes of mozzarella and salt and pepper as desired, then toss again
- Cover and leave in the fridge to chill (approx 2 hours)
- Remove 10 minutes before serving
- Finely chop the parsley, shred the basil leaves and sprinkle them over the salad
- Give the salad a final toss

Day's total: 499 calories

Menu 2

Breakfast - 170 calories

Poached eggs with Crispbread

1 cal cooking spray
2 medium eggs
Salt
Ground black pepper
2 crispbreads

- Coat a microwavable bowl with cooking spray
- Break eggs into bowl, prick yolks
- Spray eggs with cooking spray
- Add salt and pepper to taste
- Cover bowl loosely
- Microwave on high setting for 2 minutes or 1½ minutes if you prefer your yolks softer (based on 750 watt)
- Serve with crispbread slices (e.g. Ryvita)

Spicy Tomato soup

½ garlic clove, chopped
2 slices root ginger, chopped
½ green chilli, chopped
Pinch ground cumin
½ tsp ground coriander
14g (½ oz) red split lentils
200g (½ can) chopped tomatoes
300ml (10 fl.oz) vegetable stock
½ tbsp tamarind paste
A few coriander leaves
1 tbsp natural yogurt
1 cal cooking oil spray

- Cook the garlic, ginger and chilli in oil spray (about 6 sprays) for 3 minutes to blend flavours
- Add the spices and cook for a further two minutes
- Add the coriander, lentils, tomatoes and stock
- Bring to boil and stir in the tamarind paste
- Simmer for 20 minutes until the lentils are tender
- Transfer to a blender and blend until smooth
- Chop the coriander leaves and fold into the yoghurt
- Stir into the soup and serve

Dinner - 210 calories

Ham & Roasted Vegetables

2 slices cooked ham
½ tbsp olive oil
42g (1½ oz) beets, cubed
42g (1½ oz) onion, cubed
42g (1½ oz) parsnip, cubed
42g (1½ oz) turnip, cubed
42g (1½ oz) courgette (zucchini), cubed
42g (1½ oz) red pepper, cubed
Pinch salt & black pepper

- Preheat oven to 200°C / 390°F / Gas mark 6
- Place cubed vegetables into a bowl
- Sprinkle with olive oil and mix well
- Season with the salt and pepper
- Spread the vegetables out evenly on a baking tray lined with greased foil
- Roast in the hot oven for about 45 minutes, turning halfway through cooking
- Remove from oven when tender and beginning to turn golden
- Serve immediately with the ham slices

Day's total: 490 calories

Menu 3

Breakfast - 108 calories

Hot, Cold & Spicy Smoothie

1 tsp honey
½ tsp ground cinnamon
Very tiny sprinkle of hot chilli pepper
Pinch ground nutmeg
1 small banana (6 inches or less) peeled and sliced
28g (1 oz) kale, chopped
14g (½ oz) spinach
60ml (2 fl.oz) water
Ice cubes

- Mix all the above in a blender on high speed until completely smooth
- Add the ice cubes and blend thoroughly
- Pour into a glass and it's ready to drink and savour each mouthful.

Lunch – 142 calories

Tomato and Cabbage Salad with Edamame

1 teaspoon extra virgin olive oil
1 fl. oz lemon juice
8 cherry tomatoes, halved
70g (2½ oz) cabbage, chopped
56g (2 oz) ready-shelled edamame beans
4 olives, halved or sliced

- Cook the edamame beans, as per packet instructions
- Put the cooked beans into a small salad bowl and allow them to cool
- Add the cabbage, cherry tomatoes and olives to the beans
- Drizzle the olive oil and lemon juice over the salad
- Toss the salad to coat evenly

Dinner - 250 calories

Ham, Cheese & Tomato Omelette

2 medium eggs
1 teaspoon wholegrain mustard
1 cal olive oil spray
1 slice cooked ham
3 cherry tomatoes
14g (½ oz) grated cheddar cheese
Salt
Ground black pepper
Sprigs of parsley

- Cut the ham into small pieces
- Slice the cherry tomatoes in half
- Separate the egg yolks from the whites
- Beat the yolks with mustard, salt and pepper
- Whisk the egg whites until they stand in soft peaks
- Stir the whites gently into the yolks
- Heat the grill to a high temperature
- Spray an omelette pan with 6 sprays of olive oil spray
- Pour the egg mixture into the pan
- Cook over a medium heat until the underside is golden (about 2 minutes)
- Put the pan under the grill and cook until the top is golden (1 to 2 minutes)
- Sprinkle the ham, cheese and tomatoes over the omelette
- Fold the omelette in half
- Serve, garnished with the parsley

Day's total: 500 calories

Menu 4

Breakfast - 154 calories

Banana and Blackberry Smoothie

1 pot (125g) low fat natural yogurt
½ small banana
84g (3 oz) blackberries
120ml (4 fl.oz) water
Ice cubes
Stevia if desired
Mint leaf to decorate

- Blend together banana, blackberries, yoghurt and water on high speed setting until smooth
- If extra sweetness is required, stir in a little Stevia to taste and blend again for a few seconds
- Serve with ice cubes and top with the mint leaf

Lunch - 118 calories

Fig and Feta Omelette

28g (1 oz) kale, chopped
14g ((½ oz) spinach
½ small fig
½ tablespoon spring onions, chopped
28g (1 oz) aubergine (egg-plant), sliced
14g (½ oz) reduced fat feta cheese
1 cal olive oil spray
1 small egg
Pinch ground or grated nutmeg
3 large leaves from a round lettuce
Pinch salt
Ground black pepper

- Place spinach and kale in pan of boiling water and simmer for 4 minutes
- Drain thoroughly and place on kitchen towelling to absorb excess water
- Gently fry spring onion and aubergine in an omelette pan in a few sprays of oil for 3 minutes
- Remove from heat, sprinkle with nutmeg, salt and pepper
- Stir in the spinach and kale
- Pre-heat grill to medium high heat
- Whisk the egg
- Pour the egg over the mixture
- Top with feta cheese and figs. Grill until golden brown.
- Serve on a bed of lettuce

Dinner - 220 calories

Spicy Chicken with Tomato, Pepper & Mint Salad

1 small chicken breast (84g/3oz), skinless
¾ tablespoons tamarind purée
1 teaspoon root ginger, grated
¾ teaspoon chilli powder (mild)
Pinch of Stevia
8 cherry tomatoes
Couple of mint leaves, chopped
¼ green chilli, seeded and sliced
1 small sweet yellow pepper
1 small onion
1 large wedge of lemon
Salt & Pepper

- Chop the chicken into chunky pieces
- Place in a bowl and add the tamarind purée, grated ginger, half the chilli powder, pinch of Stevia and salt and pepper
- Mix well and leave to infuse for approximately ten minutes
- Preheat the grill to a high temperature
- Cut the tomatoes in half and finely slice the onion and yellow pepper
- Place the tomatoes, pepper and onion in a bowl and add the chilli, mint, the juice of the lemon wedge and the rest of the chilli powder
- Season with salt and pepper to taste
- Push the chicken pieces onto a metal skewer
- Grill the skewered chicken, turning frequently until cooked thoroughly (about ten minutes)
- Place the chicken on a plate and arrange the salad around it admiringly

Day's total: 492 calories

Menu 5

Breakfast - 127 calories

Egg & Vegetable Bake

2 large vine tomatoes, halved
1 large mushroom
¼ garlic clove, chopped finely
½ teaspoon olive oil
42g (1(½ oz) spinach
1 small egg
Salt
Black Pepper

- Heat the oven to 200^0C / 390^0F / Gas mark 6
- Put tomatoes with mushroom & garlic into an ovenproof dish
- Season with salt and pepper and pour over the oil
- Cook in the oven for 8 minutes
- While it is cooking, pour boiling water over the spinach in a colander to make it wilt
- Tip the spinach onto a piece of kitchen towel. Cover with another piece of kitchen towel and press evenly to remove any water
- After the 10 minutes of baking, remove the dish from the oven and put the spinach in with the other vegetables
- Make a small space in the middle of the vegetables and break the egg into it
- Bake for approximately 8 minutes until the egg is cooked

Lunch - 115 calories

Carrot & Coriander Soup

½ onion, chopped
¼ teaspoon ground coriander
2 new potatoes, finely diced
112g (4 oz) carrots, grated
300ml (10 fl.oz) vegetable stock
1 teaspoon coriander leaves, chopped
1 cal olive oil

- Spray a saucepan with 4 sprays 1 cal oil and heat
- Fry the onion for a few minutes until soft
- Mix in the potato and coriander and cook for a further minute
- Add in the carrots and vegetable stock, boil up then reduce heat and cover the pan
- Simmer for about 15 minutes
- Pour the mixture into a blender and add the coriander leaves
- Blend thoroughly until completely smooth
- Reheat if necessary
- Pour into a serving bowl

Dinner - 239 calories

Halibut with Barbecue Sauce

½ fillet halibut
1 tablespoon sugar-free apricot jams
½ teaspoon fresh root ginger, finely chopped
2 tablespoons orange juice
2 tablespoons lime juice
½ teaspoon strong mustard
¼ teaspoon cinnamon
¼ teaspoon nutmeg
1 cal olive oil spray
Salt
Ground black pepper

- Put all the ingredients except the fish into a saucepan and boil up
- Reduce the heat and simmer for 5 minutes
- Remove from heat
- Heat the grill to a high setting
- Place the fish on a non-stick grill pan and season with salt and pepper
- Spray fish with olive oil spray (2 sprays)
- Grill for 4 minutes, turn over and brush with the sauce
- Cook for a further 3 minutes
- Brush again with the sauce before serving

Day's total: 481 calories

Menu 6

Breakfast - 170 calories

Cheese & Tomato Omelette

1 cal olive oil
6 cherry tomatoes
½ small onion, diced
6 fresh basil leaves, chopped
2 small eggs
1 tablespoon grated Parmesan cheese
Salt
Pepper

- Coat a small pan with 5 sprays of 1 cal olive oil and heat gently
- Fry the onion until soft (approximately 4 minutes)
- At the halved tomatoes to the onion and cook for a further 2 – 3 minutes
- Remove from the heat and mix in the basil
- Whisk the eggs with a tablespoon of water and season with salt and pepper
- Heat 4 sprays of 1 cal olive oil in an omelette pan
- Pour in the egg and cook until set
- Sprinkle Parmesan cheese onto one half of the omelette and spread the tomato mixture over the cheese
- Fold the plain half of the omelette over the filled half and cook for a further two minutes until the base is golden brown
- Serve immediately and savour

Zesty Prawn and Grapefruit Salad

42g (1½ oz) fresh prawns, cooked and ready to use
1 small grapefruit, segmented
2 large leaves from a round lettuce
1 tablespoon low fat mayonnaise
A few drops of Tabasco sauce
6 fresh mint leaves, chopped
Salt
Pepper

- Spoon the mayonnaise into a cup and season with Tabasco sauce, salt and pepper to taste
- Place the salad leaves overlapping in the middle of a plate
- Arrange the prawns and grapefruit segments on centre of the lettuce
- Sprinkle the mint leaves on top
- Spoon the spicy mayonnaise onto the side of the plate to use as a dip

Dinner - 240 calories

Spicy Chicken Breast

1 skinless chicken breast fillet
2 sprigs of parsley, finely chopped
Pinch of cumin
Pinch of coriander
1 cal olive oil spray
120 ml (4 fl.oz) vegetable stock
Pepper
Pinch of chilli powder (optional)

Side salad:

56g (2 oz) lettuce
6 radishes
1 tomato quartered
6 slices cucumber

- Pre-heat oven to 200^0C / 390^0F / Gas mark 6
- Use a sharp knife to make 3 small cuts in the chicken
- In a bowl, mix the herbs and spices well
- Cover the chicken breast with the mixture, pushing some of it into the cuts
- Spray twice with the olive oil
- Pour the stock into a small, shallow oven dish
- Carefully transfer the chicken fillet onto the dish
- Cook for 20 minutes. Make sure the chicken is cooked thoroughly and that the coating is golden brown before removing
- Slice the chicken and serve with the side salad

Day's total: 497 calories

Menu7

Breakfast - 123 calories

Grape Booster

168g (6 oz) seedless grapes, red
84g (3 oz) seedless grapes, green
60ml (2 fl.oz) purple grape juice
1 teaspoon lime juice
½ teaspoon root ginger, chopped
Ice cubes

- Put the grapes, juices, ginger and ice cubes into a blender and mix thoroughly
- Serve in a tall glass

Lunch - 94 calories

Filled Mushrooms

3 large mushrooms, cleaned and hollowed out
½ tablespoon tomatoes, chopped
½ tablespoon red peppers, chopped
½ tablespoon olives, chopped
½ fresh garlic clove
¼ tablespoon fresh parsley, finely chopped
¼ teaspoon fresh oregano leaves, chopped
Fresh ground black pepper, to taste
¼ teaspoon fresh lemon juice
½ teaspoon olive oil
28g (1 oz) feta cheese, crumbled
3 sprigs parsley to garnish

- Lightly grease a baking tray or line with foil
- Clean the mushrooms with a damp piece of kitchen towel
- Remove the stalks and hollow out the heads
- Mix the tomatoes, peppers, olives, parsley, oregano, lemon and olive oil in a bowl
- Crush the garlic into the mix and stir well
- Fill the mushroom heads equally and put them on the baking tray
- Cook for approximately 20 minutes or until the smell drives you mad with anticipation
- Serve on a plate with a sprig of parsley to garnish each one

Dinner - 258 calories

Spicy Fish Dish

126g (4½ oz) fillet white fish
1 tablespoon chilli pesto
½ tablespoon breadcrumbs
½ tablespoon Parmesan cheese, grated
112g (4 oz) green beans, trimmed
½ teaspoon of butter
½ lemon, sliced in wedges
Salt
Pepper

- Heat the oven to 200^0C / 390^0F Gas mark 6
- Put the fillet on a greased baking tray
- Season with salt and pepper and coat with chilli pesto
- Mix the breadcrumbs with the Parmesan cheese and sprinkle on the fish
- Bake for about 10 minutes until the fish is cooked and the topping bubbles
- Meanwhile, boil or steam the beans until tender then stir in the butter and the juice of one lemon wedge
- Arrange the fish on a plate with the beans and decorate with the remainder of the lemon wedges

Note: adjust the amount of chilli pesto to suit your own taste. It can be quite fiery!

Day's total: 475 calories

Menu 8

Breakfast - 150 calories

Fruity Delight

1 small pot fat-free peach yogurt
84g (3 oz) pineapple chunks, canned or fresh
56g (2 oz) raspberries, fresh or frozen

Layer a sundae glass with yoghurt, pineapple and raspberries, with a raspberry on top of the yoghurt
And that's it. Easy peasy!

Lunch - 80 calories

Tasty Green Veggie Soup

3 sticks celery, chopped
¼ leek, sliced
56g (2 oz) spinach
300ml (10 fl.oz) vegetable stock
1 cal olive oil spray
½ tablespoon fat-free yoghurt

- Use 5 sprays of olive oil to coat a frying pan
- Fry the leek and celery on a gentle heat for approximately 5 minutes, until the leeks are soft
- Add the stock and cook for 25 minutes on a low heat
- Mix in the spinach and continue to cook for 5 minutes
- Pour the mixture into a blender and liquidize
- Swirl in the yoghurt and serve

Dinner - 227 calories

Beefy Chilli Stir Fry

56g (2 oz) fillet steak, thinly sliced
½ red chilli, deseeded and chopped
2 teaspoons rice wine vinegar
1 piece root ginger, finely chopped
1 clove garlic, crushed
2 teaspoons light soy sauce
2 spring onions, trimmed and sliced
112g (4 oz) broccoli, chopped into small pieces
112g (4 oz) courgettes (zucchini), diced
84g (3 oz) pak choi (Chinese cabbage), chopped
1 teaspoon sesame oil

- Stir the chilli, ginger and garlic into the soy sauce and rice wine vinegar
- Put the beef slices into the sauce mix
- Heat the sesame oil in a wok until it smokes
- Lift the beef from the sauce and cook with the courgettes and spring onion for 1 minute
- Add the broccoli and pak choi to the wok and cook for another 2 minutes, stirring continuously until cooked
- Pour in the sauce and stir well
- Serve immediately

Day's total: 457 calories

Menu 9

Breakfast - 98 calories

Pear Peach & Strawberry Cocktail

½ pear, peeled and chopped
½ peach, stoned and chopped
112g (4 oz) strawberries, halved
Large wedge of lime
Ice cube

- Put the pear. Peach and strawberries into a blender
- Squeeze the juice of the lime on top
- Add the ice cube
- Blend until smooth
- Pour into a glass and drink

Lunch - 200 calories

Honeyed Chicken Stir-Fry with Noodles

1 small skinless chicken breast
4 teaspoons sweet chilli stir fry sauce
1½ teaspoons clear honey
14g (½ oz) fresh root ginger, grated
1 clove garlic, finely chopped
1 tablespoon water
2 spring onions, trimmed and thinly sliced
28g (1 oz) precooked rice noodles
Salt
Pepper

- In a cup, mix the sweet chilli stir-fry sauce, honey, ginger, garlic and water
- Dice the chicken
- Heat a wok and dry-fry the chicken pieces for a few seconds to colour them
- Pour the honey mixture over the chicken and stir
- Season with salt and pepper
- Stir-fry over a medium heat for about 10 minutes
- Add the precooked noodles for the last 3 minutes
- Serve with the sliced spring onion scattered over the top

Dinner - 200 calories

Lemon and Parsley Haddock with Green Beans

1 fresh haddock fillet
Juice and grated zest of ½ lemon
56g (2 oz) breadcrumbs
6 sprigs parsley, finely chopped
1 tomato, halved
1 cal olive oil spray
112g (4 oz) trimmed green beans
Salt
Pepper

- Preheat the oven to 170^0C / 340^0F / Gas mark 3- 4
- Mix the breadcrumbs, lemon zest, parsley and lemon juice
- Add salt and pepper to taste
- Use the breadcrumb mix to coat the fish
- Spray a baking tray with 2 sprays 1 cal olive oil
- Put the coated fish and tomato halves on the baking tray
- Spray twice with 1 cal olive oil
- Cook in the oven for 20 minutes
- While it is cooking, steam or boil the beans
- Serve the fish with the cooked green beans

Day's total: 498 calories

Menu 10

Breakfast - 150 calories

Banana and Ginger Smoothie

1 extra small banana (below 6 inches)
¼ teaspoon ginger root, grated
1 tablespoon coconut milk
60ml (2 fl.oz) apple juice
Ice cubes

- Put all the ingredients in a blender
- Blend thoroughly
- Serve in a glass

Lunch - 127 calories

Courgette (zucchini) and Chive Omelette

2 small eggs
1 courgette (zucchini), finely diced
1 teaspoon chives, chopped
1 cal olive oil
Salt
Pepper

- Whisk the eggs thoroughly
- Add the courgette and chives
- Season with salt and pepper
- Spray a frying pan with 3 sprays olive oil and heat on a medium setting
- Pour in the egg mixture
- Cook until firm on one side then flip over and cook until the base is golden brown
- Serve immediately

Dinner - 180 calories

Chilli Chicken Stir Fry

84g (3 oz) chicken breast strips, skinless
1 tablespoon spicy chipotle chilli paste
154g (5 ½ oz) vegetable stir fry mix
1 cal olive oil spray

- Mix the chipotle chilli paste thoroughly with the chicken strips
- Leave to marinate for 1 hour
- Spray a wok with 2 sprays of olive oil and fry the chicken, stirring continuously for 3 to 5 minutes until completely cooked
- Remove the chicken and place on one side
- Spray the wok with 2 more sprays of oil
- Stir fry the vegetable mix for about 2 minutes on a medium heat
- Stir in the chicken whilst heating for a further 3 minutes
- Serve up!

Note: as with any chilli product, the chilli paste should be adjusted to your own taste. It can be quite fiery!

Days total: 457 calories

Menu 11

Breakfast - 130 calories

Spicy Apple Porridge

1 small apple, cubed
1 teaspoon vanilla essence
1 teaspoon cinnamon
A pinch of mixed spice
1 teaspoon raisins
60ml (2 fl.oz) water
10g ($^1/_3$ oz) porridge oats
60ml (2 fl.oz) semi-skimmed milk
Stevia to taste (optional)

- Place the cubed apples in a pan with the vanilla essence, cinnamon, mixed spice, raisins and ¼ cup of water
- Put the lid on the pan and simmer, stirring occasionally for about 10 minutes
- Remove from heat and leave covered
- Mix the oats with the semi-skimmed milk and salt in a large, microwavable bowl
- Cook on full power for 2 minutes
- Pour the porridge into a serving bowl and add the stewed, spicy apple. Leave in the centre or swirl in gently
- Sweeten with Stevia to taste

Lunch – 179 calories

Salmon and Cream Cheese Toasty Munch

1 slice wholemeal bread
1 tablespoon low-fat cream cheese

28g (1 oz) sliced smoked salmon
1 small red onion, sliced
56g (2 oz) alfalfa and radish shoots

- Toast the bread on both sides
- Spread the cream cheese on top of the toast
- Arrange the salmon, onions slices and alfalfa & radish shoots over the top
- Eat and enjoy!

Dinner – 191 calories

Vegetable Stir Fry

1 cal olive oil spray
4 spring onions, thinly sliced
1 tablespoon root ginger, chopped finely
½ small yellow pepper, sliced thinly
½ small red pepper, sliced thinly
1 leaf choi sum., shredded
56g (2 oz) bean sprouts
1 clove garlic, chopped
56g (2 oz) sugar snaps peas
1 tablespoon sesame oil
2 tablespoons soy sauce

- Coat a wok well with olive oil spray 6 sprays
- Fry the onions, ginger and garlic gently until soft (about 3 minutes)
- Add the peppers and sugar snap peas and continue cooking for 3 more minutes
- Add the choi sum and bean sprouts, together with the soy sauce and sesame oil
- Stir fry for a further 2 minutes
- Serve straight away

Day's total: 500 calories

Menu 12

Breakfast - 108 calories

Poached Egg with Watercress and Tomatoes

1 large egg
6 cherry tomatoes, diced
28g (1oz) watercress, chopped
1 tsp sunflower seeds
1 teaspoon coriander, chopped

- Boil a small pan of water
- Remove from heat and swirl the water rapidly with a wooden spoon
- Break the egg into the centre of the swirling water
- Cook for about two minutes or until the egg is firm
- Remove egg with a slotted spoon and allow the water to drain away
- Place the sunflower seeds dry into a heavy-bottomed pan or skillet
- Heat over a medium heat for about 2 minutes or until golden brown, keeping the pan moving to avoid burning the seeds
- Mix the seeds with the watercress and tomatoes and arrange on a plate
- Place the egg on the salad and top with coriander

Lunch - 112 calories

Potato, Onion & Greens Soup

¼ bunch spring onions, chopped
1 cal olive oil spray
1 small potato, peeled and diced
300ml (10 fl.oz) vegetable stock
70g (2½ oz) watercress, spinach and rocket (arugula) salad
Pepper
Sprig of parsley
Slice of crispbread

- Coat the bottom of a small saucepan with 5 sprays of 1 cal olive oil spray and heat
- Fry the chopped spring onions gently until tender
- Put in the potato and cook with the onions for 2 minutes
- Pour in the stock, add a little black pepper and cook until the potato is soft and beginning to crumble
- Stir in the salad leaves and continue to cook gently for a further minute
- Pour into a blender and liquidize thoroughly
- Serve, topped with a sprig of parsley
- Enjoy with a crispbread slice

Dinner - 270 calories

Grilled Lamb Chop Special

2 lamb loin chops (about 190g - 7 oz - total)
¼ of small orange pepper, diced
1 teaspoon chopped red onion
28g (1 oz) baby spinach leaves
Wedge of lemon
1 cal olive oil spray

Dressing:
    ¼ teaspoon grated lemon rind
    1 tablespoon clear honey
    ¼ tablespoon fresh thyme, chopped
    ¼ clove garlic, finely chopped
    ½ teaspoon grain mustard
    Salt
    Ground pepper

- Preheat the grill to a medium level
- Put the dressing ingredients into a medium sized bowl and mix well
- Remove 1 teaspoon of the dressing and put in a salad bowl for later
- Coat the chops thoroughly in the bowl with the remainder of the dressing and leave to marinate for about 10 minutes
- Spray the grill pan with 3 sprays of olive oil
- Place the chops on the grill pan
- Grill gently, turning occasionally until cooked to your taste (about 10 minutes for medium rare)
- In the bowl with the teaspoon of dressing put the orange pepper, onion and spinach leaves and mix well
- Put the dressed salad on a plate and place the chops on top
- Put the lemon wedge on the side of the plate and your delicious meal is ready.

Day's total: 490 calories

Menu 13

Breakfast - 75 calories

Fruit & Vegetable Juice

½ medium carrot
2 sticks celery
1 apple
1 tomato
1 thin slice root ginger
Sprig of mint

- Cut all ingredients except mint into small pieces
- Put pieces into juicer and switch on
- Collect the juice in a glass
- Pop in the sprig of mint
- Done!

Lunch - 183 calories

Chicken Liver Lunch

56g (2 oz) chicken liver
112g (4 oz) green beans
¼ teaspoon olive oil
4 thin spring onions, sliced

For the Dressing:

1 tsp olive oil
1 tbsp soy sauce
½ teaspoon cider vinegar

- Steam the green beans until tender.
- Meanwhile, preheat the grill on a medium setting
- Press the liver flat and place on a grill tray
- Drizzle ¼ tsp olive oil over the liver
- Grill the liver for 2 minutes on each side
- Mix the ingredients for the dressing in a small bowl
- Stir in the spring onion and beans
- Slice the liver finely and stir into the salad
- Spoon onto a plate and eat

Dinner - 225 calories

Mediterranean Beef

84g (3 oz) lean beef steak, thinly sliced
¼ garlic clove, sliced
¼ onion, sliced
1 cal olive oil spray
100g (3½ oz) canned chopped tomatoes
¼ yellow pepper, thinly sliced

Pinch chopped rosemary
2 olives, chopped
84g (3 oz) slice of precooked polenta

- Spray a saucepan with 4 sprays olive oil
- Fry the onion and garlic for about 5 minutes until the onion is starting to brown
- Add the beef, tomatoes, pepper and rosemary and stir well
- Simmer gently in the covered pan, stirring occasionally, until the beef is cooked (about 15 minutes)
- Preheat the grill to medium
- If the mixture becomes too dry, add a little boiling water
- Add the olives and stir again
- Grill the polenta for about 3 minutes each side during the last six minutes of the beef cooking
- Place the polenta beside the beef mix on a plate and serve hot. Buona appetita!

Day's total: 483 calories

Menu 14

Breakfast - 128 calories

Pineapple and Cottage Cheese Toasty

1 slice wholemeal bread
28g (1 oz) cottage cheese
1 teaspoon cinnamon
1 slice pineapple

- Preheat the grill to a medium heat
- Toast the bread lightly on both sides
- Spread the cottage cheese evenly over the toast
- Sprinkle with the cinnamon
- Place the pineapple on top
- Put the toasty under the grill
- Grill until the cheese begins to brown

Lunch - 159 calories

Greek Salad

1 plum tomato, chopped
28g (1 oz) low fat feta cheese
½ small yellow pepper, chopped
½ red onion, chopped
¼ cucumber, diced
3 large pitted olives, halved

Dressing:
  ½ tablespoon balsamic vinegar
  ¼ tablespoon olive oil
  Salt & ground black pepper

- Place all the prepared salad vegetables in a bowl
- Crumble the feta cheese into the salad
- Pour the vinegar and olive oil into a small lidded container, add a small amount of salt and pepper and shake vigorously
- Pour the dressing onto the salad and mix well before serving

Note: if you increase the quantities of the dressing you can store the remainder in the fridge for another salad on another day.

Dinner - 188 calories

Baked Vegetables with Salmon

1 salmon fillet
1 very small garlic clove, crushed
1 tablespoon extra virgin olive oil
½ small tomato, chopped
28g (1 oz) spinach
70g (2½ oz) mushrooms, chopped
3 large leaves from a round lettuce

- Preheat the oven to 190° C / 375° F / Gas mark 5
- Use a little of the olive oil to grease a small baking dish
- Place the salmon on the baking dish, skin underneath
- Put the rest of the olive oil into a small bowl, add the garlic, tomato, spinach and mushrooms, and mix thoroughly
- Cover the salmon with the mixture
- Cook for about 20 minutes
- Serve on a bed of lettuce

Day's total: 475 calories

Menu 15

Breakfast - 136 calories

Scrummy Scrambled Egg

1 large egg
1 tablespoon water
42g (1½ oz) onion, chopped
1 small firm tomato, diced
4 good sized basil leaves, chopped finely
2 tablespoons grated low fat cheddar cheese
Salt to taste
Ground pepper to taste
1 cal olive oil spray
2 sprigs fresh parsley

- Beat egg and water in a bowl
- Coat a small frying pan with 4 sprays of 1 cal spray and heat
- Add onion and cook gently whilst stirring until soft and translucent
- Mix in the diced tomato, chopped basil leaves, salt and pepper
- Cook for a further minute
- Pour the beaten egg into the pan and stir continuously until the egg is cooked
- Transfer to a plate scatter with the grated cheese
- Decorate with the parsley and savour slowly!

Lunch - 185 calories

Tuna Salad

½ small can tuna chunks in brine
1 large egg
4 cherry tomatoes, halved
3 large lettuce leaves, shredded
Salt
Pepper

- Hard-boil the egg in boiling water (about 10 minutes). Drain and leave to cool
- Put the shredded lettuce and the tomatoes in a bowl with the tuna and mix together
- When the egg has cooled down, shell and chop it
- Stir the egg pieces into the rest of the salad
- Season and serve

Dinner - 179 calories

Chicken & Mushroom Broth, Thai Style

56g (2 oz) ready cooked chicken, shredded
240ml (8 fl.oz) chicken stock
¼ tablespoon Thai red curry paste
¼ tablespoon Thai fish sauce
½ lime, zest and juice
½ teaspoon sugar
28g (1 oz) mushrooms, sliced
2 spring onions, chopped

- Heat the stock in a medium sized saucepan
- Add the curry paste, sugar, fish sauce, lime juice and zest
- When boiling, add in the mushrooms and spring onion pieces
- Cover the pan and simmer the mixture for 2 minutes
- Add the chicken and stir well
- Serve in your favourite bowl

Day's total: 500 calories

Menu16

Breakfast - 209 calories

Tropical Shake

126g (4½ oz) tropical fruit, frozen
1 tablespoon oats
100ml (3½ fl.oz) orange juice
100ml (3½ fl.oz) soya milk

- Put all the ingredients into a blender
- Blend thoroughly until completely smooth
- Serve in a tall glass

Lunch - 69 calories

Hot Toddy

½ lemon
Small piece fresh root ginger, finely sliced
3 teaspoons honey
300 ml (10 fl.oz) boiling water

- Cut the lemon into two pieces and squeeze the juice of one piece into a mug
- Cut the other piece of lemon into slices
- Put the lemon slices, ginger and honey in the mug
- Add the boiling water
- Allow 5 minutes for infusion
- It's ready to drink. Cheers!

If you have a cold, this drink is very soothing. If you don't, it's delicious anyway.

Dinner - 203 calories

Mediterranean Chicken

112g (4 oz) diced chicken breast
½ garlic clove, sliced
100g (3½ oz) rocket (arugula)
2 sticks celery, finely chopped
1 teaspoon basil, chopped
½ lemon
¼ onion, chopped
6 cherry tomatoes, halved
1 cal olive oil

- Spray a frying pan with 3 sprays of olive oil
- Fry the chicken gently until cooked (about 10 minutes) and turn off the heat
- Put the garlic, rocket, celery, basil and onion into a blender and squeeze in the lemon juice
- Blend thoroughly
- Pour the mixture over the chicken, add the tomatoes and stir well
- Serve while hot

Day's total: 481

Menu 17

Breakfast - 163 calories

Toasty Spicy Slice

1 slice of white bread
1 teaspoon peanut butter
1 tablespoon natural fat-free yoghurt
1 small banana, sliced
Small pinch of cinnamon
Small pinch of ground ginger
Small pinch of mixed spice

- Mix the peanut butter and yoghurt thoroughly in a bowl
- Toast the bread
- Spread the mixture on the toast and arrange the slices of banana on top
- Season with the cinnamon, ginger and mixed spice
- Eat slowly, relishing each mouthful

Lunch - 120 calories

Smoked Salmon and Radishes with Poppy Seed Dressing

56g (2 oz) smoked salmon
¼ tablespoon poppy seeds
Juice and zest of ½ orange
½ teaspoon cider vinegar
½ teaspoon olive oil
A couple of drops of sesame oil
8 radishes, finely sliced
1 spring onion, finely sliced
Black pepper
1 slice of crispbread

- In a bowl, mix thoroughly the poppy seeds, vinegar, sesame oil, olive oil, orange zest and juice and black pepper
- Place the salmon in another bowl and add the sliced radishes and spring onion
- Pour the dressing over the salmon and mix everything carefully until the salmon is completely coated
- Leave to marinate for 10 minutes
- Place the salmon on a plate and pour over any remaining dressing
- Serve up with two slices of crispbread

Dinner - 206 calories

Chicken Tandoori

2 small chicken thighs, skinless
Juice of ¼ lemon
½ tsp paprika
½ red onion, finely chopped
1 cal olive oil
1 garlic & coriander poppadom (accompaniment)

Marinade:

    56g (2 oz) fat-free Greek yogurt
    Pinch ground cumin
    Small piece of ginger, grated
    Pinch garam masala
    ½ garlic clove, crushed
    Pinch chilli powder
    Pinch turmeric

- In a bowl, mix together the paprika, lemon juice and onion
- With a sharp knife make 2 slits in each chicken thigh
- Coat the thighs well with the juice and leave them in the bowl to steep for 10 minutes
- Take a jug, put all the marinade ingredients into it, and stir thoroughly
- Pour the marinade onto the chicken thighs and coat them well with the mixture
- Cover the bowl and refrigerate for 1 hour
- Heat the grill to medium
- Put the chicken pieces on a lightly oiled baking tray and spray a couple of times with the olive oil
- Grill them for 8 minutes before turning over and grilling the other side for a further 8 minutes
- Check that the chicken is thoroughly cooked before serving
- Serve with the poppadom

Day's total: 489 calories

Menu 18

Breakfast - 130 calories

Sharp and Sweet Fruit Salad

½ tablespoon lemon juice
1 small apple, cubed
84g (3 oz) strawberries, chopped
70g (2½ oz) canned mandarin orange segments in juice
56g (2 oz) canned grapefruit segments in juice
Stevia to taste (optional)

- Put the apple and strawberries into a serving bowl and coat well with the lemon juice
- Stir in the grapefruit and mandarin segments with their juice
- If the flavour is too sharp for your taste, add a little Stevia

Note: Leaving the cans of grapefruit and mandarin in the fridge overnight will chill them nicely for a refreshing summer breakfast.

Lunch - 87 calories

Cauliflower and Onion Soup

300ml (10 fl.oz) vegetable stock
1 tablespoon lemon juice
1 small cauliflower, separated into florets
1 cal olive oil
6 spring onions, trimmed & chopped
Small pinch nutmeg
Large pinch black pepper
Sprig of parsley

- Put the stock and lemon juice in a pan and heat until boiling

- Lower the heat to medium and cook the cauliflower in the liquid for 8 to 10 minutes until soft
- Cover and leave
- Heat the oil in a frying pan on a medium heat and fry the chopped onions for 4 – 5 minutes
- Stir the cooked spring onions into the pan with the cauliflower
- Pour the contents of the pan into a blender and blend until smooth
- Add the pepper and nutmeg and stir
- Serve with a garnish of parsley

Dinner - 276 calories

Courgette (zucchini), Lentil and Feta Salad

500g (18 oz) baby courgettes (zucchini)
1 tsp olive oil
2 tablespoons cooked puy lentils (canned)
28g (1 oz) feta cheese, cut into small chunks
¾ teaspoon lemon zest
1 tablespoon mint leaves, shredded
Pinch of salt

- Cut the courgettes lengthwise into long batons
- Put them on a plate, add a pinch of salt and turn well until all the batons are oily
- Place the batons onto a hot, ridged griddle
- Cook until the batons have brown stripes on both sides. Turn while cooking
- Place the courgettes in a bowl and add the lentils, feta cheese and lemon zest
- Mix thoroughly
- Stir in the shredded mint leaves and serve

Day's total: 493 calories

Menu 19

Breakfast - 150 calories

Banana Muffins

112g (4 oz) self-raising flour
Generous pinch of salt
1 medium banana, mashed
28g (1 oz) sugar
28g (1 oz) apple sauce
1 small egg
A few drops of vanilla essence

- Preheat oven to 170^0C / 350^0F / Gas mark 3-4
- Grease muffin tray or muffin cups
- Put flour and salt into a mixing bowl
- Into another bowl, place the mashed banana, sugar, vanilla and egg and beat well, then stir in the apple sauce
- Scoop the banana mixture into the flour and mix well
- Divide the mixture evenly into six muffin cups
- Place in the oven and bake for 20 minutes. If a toothpick pushed into the centre emerges clean, the muffins are cooked
- Allow to cool before eating
- Eat two and store the rest

This recipe makes 6 muffins. The rest may be stored in an airtight storage box. The flavour improves overnight so making them the night before will mean you have a ready breakfast when you get up.

Refreshing Raspberry Fizz

84g (3 oz) raspberries
250 ml (8 fl.oz) sparkling water
Small wedge of lemon
1 teaspoon honey

- Wash raspberries and liquidize them in a blender.
- Pour into a jug and add the sparkling water and squeeze in the lemon juice.
- Stir gently.
- Sieve the mixture to get rid of seeds.
- Stir in the honey.

Dinner - 290 calories

Salmon fishcake with Petits Pois
(Makes 4 fishcakes - refrigerate three and eat one)

112g (4 oz) smoked salmon
500g (18 oz) potatoes (floury, e.g. Maris Piper)
4 spring onions
1 medium egg
1 tablespoon light mayonnaise
2 tablespoons fresh chopped parsley
1 sprig parsley for garnish
Salt to taste
Ground black pepper
5 drops Tabasco sauce (optional)
14g (½ oz) butter
56g (2 oz) breadcrumbs

- Peel and boil the potatoes until soft.
- Finely chop the salmon.
- Trim and chop the spring onions.
- Drain the potatoes and return them to the pan.
- Mash the potatoes thoroughly and mix in the spring onions.
- Put the mixture into a large bowl and spread it so that it cools quickly.
- Separate the egg and beat the yolk and mayonnaise into the mash.
- Fold in the salmon and parsley then add the seasonings.
- Divide the mixture into four equal parts and shape into fishcakes.
- Beat the egg white then brush it over the fishcakes before coating them in breadcrumbs.
- Melt the butter in a small frying pan on a medium heat and cook one fishcake gently until golden and crispy (about 5 minutes each side).
- Serve with ½ cup of cooked frozen petits pois

Day's total: 500 calories

Menu 20

Breakfast - 145 calories

Boiled Egg with Asparagus Fingers

1 large egg
1 cal olive oil spray
14g (½ oz) dried breadcrumbs
Pinch of chilli powder
Pinch of paprika
4 asparagus spears
Salt

- Fry the breadcrumbs gently in 4 sprays of hot oil until golden blown
- Mix in the chilli, paprika and salt and place to one side
- Place the asparagus in a saucepan of boiling water, add a little salt and cook until tender (about 5 minutes)
- While the asparagus is cooking, cook the egg in a pan of boiling water for approximately 5 minutes
- Put the egg in an egg cup in the middle of a plate and arrange the drained asparagus around it
- Sprinkle the crumbs over the asparagus and your breakfast is ready

Lunch - 168 calories

Minty Pineapple and Grapefruit

126g (4½ oz) pineapple rings, drained
140g (5 oz) canned red grapefruit, drained
1 tablespoon soft brown sugar
1 tablespoons mint leaves

- Arrange the fruit tastefully in a serving bowl
- Pound the mint and sugar together using a mortar and pestle
- Once they are completely blended, sprinkle the minty sugar over the fruit and enjoy the mingled flavours

Dinner - 181 calories

Vegetable Chilli

½ clove garlic, crushed
½ red chilli, chopped
¼ teaspoon ground cumin
70g (2½ oz) mushrooms, quartered
100g (3½ oz) canned kidney beans
100g (3½ oz) canned chopped tomatoes
42g (1½ oz) green beans, trimmed and sliced
50ml (1½ fl.oz) water
1 teaspoon low-fat crème fraîche
Piece of crusty bread
1 cal olive oil spray

- Spray a frying pan four times with the olive oil and heat
- Put in the garlic and the chilli and fry for 2 minutes
- Add the mushrooms and cumin and cook for a further 3 minutes

- Pour in the tomatoes, kidney beans and water
- Simmer for 10 minutes, stirring occasionally
- Mix in the green beans and cook for five more minutes until the sauce thickens and the beans are soft
- Pour into a serving bowl, top with crème fraîche and enjoy with 2 slices of crispy wheat crispbreads

Day's total: 494 calories

Chapter 6

Emily's Simple Healthy Single-Serving Smoothie Recipes

Introduction

One of the most effective ways I found to add variety to my two diet days a week was by experimenting with different types of smoothies.

They are a great way of packing healthy nutrients into a tasty drink, and can also be surprisingly filling.

They are perfect for any meal, whether it be to give you the boost you need in the morning, to keep you going throughout the day or to help you relax in the evening.

Having always previously thought of smoothies as fruit-based drinks, I was pleasantly surprised to discover that actually there are many other foods that work just as well.

In fact, something that became very quickly apparent was that often it was the really unexpected combinations that ended up with the most delicious drinks, as you will find in some of the recipes that follow.

The most common question people ask when it comes to making smoothies is whether you will need a juicer. This is really down to personal choice. You may wish to juice harder fruits and vegetables, such as apples and carrots; however, for simplicity, I use pre-packaged juice from the supermarket/grocery store.

However, I prefer juices not made from concentrates as the process they go through in the making destroys or diminishes many nutrients. So I look for ones that are labelled 'not from concentrate' or 'freshly squeezed'.

You will, however, need a blender (I've tried using the lawnmower instead and it's far too messy!).

If you are really serious about making smoothies, it's worth investing in a good quality one (blender, that is, not lawnmower), with a large, easy-to-clean jug, a heavy base to keep it steady when in use and a multi-speed motor.

The highest speed will be necessary for crushing ice and breaking down hard foods such as celery and carrot. If it is equipped with a pulse control, so much the better: among other things, this feature helps to dislodge any lumps of food that may get stuck beneath the blades, as well as giving you an extra degree of control over the whole process of preparing a smoothie.

This is not the place to get into technicalities but if you don't already own a blender I would recommend doing a bit of research online before buying one: there are plenty of websites with helpful guidance and it's worth noting that it's not always the most expensive ones that do the best job!

A citrus squeezer also comes in handy for your oranges, lemons and limes.

All the recipes are designed for a single serving. Obviously, if you do wish to make any more than this you can simply scale the amounts up accordingly. I have also listed calorie counts for each recipe in order to help you pick the smoothie that fits in best with any other meal/s you may have planned for the day.

Over time I have developed a passion for smoothie making and I am sharing with you some of my favourites.

I have tried my hardest to be as accurate as possible with measurements based on the ones I have used. However, the great thing is that there is no exact science when it comes to making smoothies and therefore do feel free to adjust any of the amounts listed according to taste (making sure to also take into account any differences in calories if you do this!).

In case you are puzzled by the use of the words 'blend', 'whizz' and 'blitz' in the recipe instructions and wonder what the difference is between them, I ought to explain that there is no difference at all. Having started by using the word 'blend' repeatedly I thought maybe the reader would prefer a bit of variety (and it made it more interesting for me, too!).

Practically Speaking

In order to help you get the most out of this section, I'm taking the liberty of adding a few practical hints. I hope you'll forgive me if some of them seem obvious but in my experience it's often the obvious that gets overlooked.

It should, for instance, go without saying that having everything you need at the ready before you start on a recipe can make life much easier and get things done faster and more tidily. But sadly, not all of us are as well organised as we should be (the voice of personal experience again!), so it's worth mentioning a basic list of items that you will need for most of the recipes and that could be kept together for ease of finding them when you need them.

The main one (and because of its size, the hardest to mislay) is your aforementioned blender. Also on your list will be a sharp knife, a measuring jug and a small measuring glass (or even a medicine pot) for measuring out smaller amounts of liquid. And don't forget the citrus squeezer. A teaspoon and a tablespoon are important items or, better still, a set of measuring spoons actually made for the purpose: I have a set that measures out one tablespoon, one teaspoon, half a teaspoon and a quarter of a teaspoon. You'll still need a proper spoon for scooping out the insides of some fruit such as papaya and kiwi.

As I said earlier, there are no fixed rules to smoothie-making; but calorie-counting is an important consideration and it's helpful in this respect to be able to measure accurately (though I hope not obsessively!).

Although some people may prefer to use a juicer to extract the juice from hard fruit and vegetables, being someone who hates having to clean two appliances when one will do, I have found that there are ways round this (some of us will go to no end of trouble to find the easy way to do something!).

One is to chop anything hard into very small chunks to make sure the blades can process them. To this end I bought a very useful gadget of the type often seen demonstrated on TV shopping channels: a multi-purpose device with a variety of blades set into the lid of a plastic box and which does everything from grating and slicing to chopping potatoes into the right size for making French fries. It's ideal for making small carrot batons and for chopping firm apples into little bits. The only downside to this wonderful device is the potential to slice fingers as well, as I found out when I first bought it. So if you buy one, please handle it more carefully than I did!

The other way to process fruit like apples and pears is to use them only when they are very ripe and soft. Pears in particular produce lovely juice when they are soft, whereas for eating purposes you'd probably prefer them firmer.

In the recipes that follow, I haven't mentioned the repetitive tasks such as washing all fruit and vegetables, taking the stones out of peaches or peeling bananas. That *would* be patronising!

Of course, your main reason for reading this section is, I'm sure, to be able use smoothies as part of your reduced-calorie days. To make this as easy as possible I have arranged all the recipes in ascending order of calorie values (i.e. lowest first).

Each smoothie has its calorie count clearly displayed after the list of ingredients. They range from 65 calories up to 246.

The idea is that you can use these smoothies to fit in with the way you intend to follow the 5:2 diet. For instance, you may prefer to have two meals rather than three on your low calorie days. In that case, having decided what to eat for your main meal, chosen perhaps from Polly's menu plans or one of Lucy's recipes, and having worked out the calorie content, you could then select a smoothie for your other meal that would make up the rest (or nearly the rest) of your allowance.

If you have planned three meals for each low-calorie day, you could do the same, adding the values of the two other meals together and supplementing them with a smoothie to make up the shortfall.

Because tastes differ, I've tried to cater for as wide a range as possible, from very sweet to spicy and savoury. And to make it even easier for you to experiment without losing track of the calories, you can refer to the calorie chart so that you can 'mix and match' armed with facts and figures.

When I started making smoothies, I kept visiting the market or supermarket for fresh fruit on an almost daily basis. But having gone through the messy job of slicing up a mango and wondering whether I didn't have anything better to do with my time, I started buying frozen fruit. This has pretty much the same calorie count, tastes just as good, is easier to control the amounts you want, saves adding ice and leaves much less mess to clear up.

Fresh and frozen fruit are for practical purposes interchangeable as far as smoothies are concerned. But if mango-slicing is your thing, don't let me stop you.

Sometimes I freeze freshly-bought fruit such as bananas and oranges to use in smoothies at a later date. The skin of a banana turns black on freezing but this in no way impairs the flesh, which becomes very creamy on being defrosted (it's best to peel them before they are completely defrosted for ease of handling). The freezing process seems to make oranges give up their juice more readily after defrosting. Grapes also freeze well and can be used instead of ice cubes.

Occasionally a recipe calls for half or less of a fruit. What can you do with the rest of it (apart, that is, from cheating and eating it!)?

One very good way to use it is to cut it into appropriately sized pieces to use as the basis for a fruit salad the next day. To avoid banana or apple slices turning brown, sprinkle them with a little lemon juice and refrigerate them.

When it comes to almond milk, rice milk and soya milk, I realise that almond, rice and soya are not mammals and that their products are therefore not, technically speaking, milk. However, milk is the name by which they're generally known so that is how I refer to them.

If you find a smoothie that sounds good to you but is too high in calories for your needs, try substituting the liquid for something such as for almond milk or coconut water, both of which have a very low calorie content (and of course there's water, which is zero-calorie rated). Or simply use a little less of an ingredient.

These measures will, obviously, change the taste but I've found that in smoothie-making, most of the liquids in these recipes combine well with all the fruit and most of the vegetables. And it's fun experimenting!

Although many of these recipes require a tall glass for serving, some produce less liquid, which looks better in a smaller glass. Filling a small glass, instead of having a half empty tall one, has the psychological effect of enjoying a larger drink. It may be an optical illusion but it definitely feels much more satisfying.

Smoothies are often thought of as a 'holiday' drink, bought at places such as tropical beach bars, so why not make the most of yours by embellishing it with a little umbrella, a very wide straw and a wedge of orange, lemon or lime?

You could also sit outdoors to drink it (though if the weather is up to its usual perverse tricks you may prefer to sit indoors and look at a picture of a tropical beach).

There is a full index of all smoothies in the Reference section at the end of this book.

I hope you enjoy these smoothies as much as I do and wish you every success eating the 5:2 way.

May your dieting go smoothie!

Cool Tomato and Cucumber

120ml (4 fl.oz) tomato juice
4 tablespoons fat-free natural yoghurt
112g (4 oz) peeled cucumber
Ice
Mint leaves

65 calories

Pour tomato juice into blender
Spoon in yoghurt
Chop and add cucumber
Add ice
Blend on high setting
Garnish with mint to serve

*Made up mostly of water, cucumbers keep the body
hydrated and help rid our bodies of toxins. Hydrating the
skin around your eyes means fewer lines and wrinkles in
the future so cut off a couple of thick slices and relax
with them over your eyes for 10 minutes whilst you sip
your smoothie*

Cranberry and Ginger

84g (3 oz) cranberries
¼ teaspoon ground ginger
240ml (8fl.oz) coconut water
Stevia to taste
Ice

65 calories

Put cranberries into blender
Add ground ginger
Pour in coconut water
Add stevia as desired
Pop in ice
Blitz thoroughly

*Cranberries are rich in vitamin C with very good
infection-fighting properties*

Fruity Fizz

180ml (6 fl.oz) sparkling water
56g (2 oz) frozen mango slices
56g (2 oz) frozen peach slices
½ apricot, canned
2 mint leaves

66 calories

Pour sparkling water into blender
Carefully add mango and peach slices
Put in apricot
Whizz thoroughly
Garnish with mint before serving

Peaches are naturally sweet and the Chinese say that their potassium content prolongs life (but still take care when crossing the road!)

Mango, Carrot and Pineapple with Citrus

28g (1 oz) frozen mango chunks
30ml (1 fl.oz) fresh orange juice
30ml (1 fl.oz) carrot juice
30ml (1 fl.oz) pineapple juice
15ml (1 tablespoon) fresh lemon juice
60ml (2 fl.oz) sparkling mineral water
½ teaspoon clear honey

75 calories

Put mango chunks into blender
Pour in the juices and mineral water
Add honey
Blend on a high setting

The beta-carotene in mango promotes glowing skin and healthy eyesight

Watercress with Fruit

14g (½ oz) watercress
42g (1½ oz) pineapple chunks
42g (1½ oz) blueberries
½ small banana
150ml (5 fl.oz) water

87 calories

Put watercress into blender.
Add all the fruit
Pour in water
Combine thoroughly in blender

Watercress is an excellent source of vitamin K which helps to strengthen bones

Creamy Rhubarb

120ml (4 fl.oz) natural fat-free yoghurt
2 ripe rhubarb stalks
1 tablespoon orange juice
Stevia to taste
60ml (2 fl.oz) water
Ice cubes

94 calories

Spoon yoghurt into blender
Chop and add rhubarb
Pour in orange juice
Add stevia as desired
Pour in water
Add ice cubes
Whizz on high setting until smooth

*The red colour in rhubarb is due to the antioxidant in it
which helps to prevent disease by giving your immune
system a boost*

Almondberry

120ml (4 fl.oz) of almond milk
4 tablespoons natural fat-free yoghurt
84g (3 oz) frozen mixed berries
½ small carrot

96 calories

Pour milk into blender
Spoon in yoghurt
Add berries
Peel, chop and add carrot
Blend until completely smooth

Almond milk is low in calories, full of vitamins and
minerals and tastes great

Fruit Sparkler

56g (2 oz) orange sorbet
56g (2 oz) fresh strawberries
56g (2 oz) canned pineapple chunks
120ml (4 fl.oz) sparkling mineral water

102 calories

Scoop sorbet into blender
Halve strawberries and add to blender
Put in pineapple chunks
Pour in water
Blend until combined

*Pineapple is a good source of fibre but low in calories,
sodium, saturated fats and cholesterol which makes it an
ideal weight loss food*

Melon, Mint and Beetroot

168g (6 oz) fresh watermelon, cubed
240ml (8 fl.oz) almond milk
6 mint leaves
4 beet leaves
A few ice cubes

107 calories

Place watermelon in blender
Pour in almond milk
Add mint, beet leaves and ice
Whizz until smooth

The fibre in beetroot leaves increases the amount of good cholesterol (HDL) in our bodies and so helps to prevent heart disease

Veggie Smoothie

120ml (4 fl.oz) low fat natural yoghurt
½ tablespoon onion
1 small stick of celery
1 medium tomato
½ cucumber
Couple of drops Tabasco Sauce
Salt and Pepper

107 calories

Spoon yoghurt into blender
Chop onion and celery finely and add
Slice and add tomato
Peel, chop and add cucumber
Shake in a couple of drops of Tabasco according to taste
Add salt and pepper
Blend until everything is combined

An accident happened to my brother Jim
When somebody threw a tomato at him
Tomatoes are juicy and don't hurt the skin
But this one was specially packed in a tin

Fibre Filler

180ml (6 fl.oz) almond milk
½ orange
½ lemon
½ peach
2 spinach leaves
1 carrot

111 calories

Pour almond milk into blender
Peel, chop and deseed lemon and orange and add
Slice peach and add
Pop in spinach leaves
Peel, slice and add carrot
Whizz until smoothly blended

*Every citrus fruit contains fibre which helps you feel
fuller for longer*

Coffee Perk

120ml (4 fl.oz) skimmed milk
60ml (2 fl.oz) strong brewed coffee
½ teaspoon instant coffee
120ml (4 fl.oz) vanilla yoghurt
¼ teaspoon vanilla essence

112 calories

Pour milk and brewed coffee into blender
Add instant coffee
Put in yoghurt and vanilla essence
Combine in blender

*Coffee contains minerals like magnesium and chromium
which help the body use insulin – the hormone that
controls blood sugar*

Parsley, Cranberry and Blueberry

¼ cucumber
120 ml (4 (fl.oz) cranberry juice
10g ($^1/_3$ oz) parsley
84g (3oz) blueberries
Stevia to taste (if you have a sweet tooth)
Ice

117 calories

Peel, chop and put cucumber into blender
Pour in cranberry juice
Chop and add parsley
Blend well
Add blueberries, ice and stevia if desired
Blend again until completely combined

Parsley contains lots of vitamin K which is important for prevention of cardiovascular disease and strokes

Blueberry-Banana Soya Heaven

240ml (8 fl.oz) soya milk
56g (2 oz) frozen blueberries
½ banana
½ teaspoon vanilla essence
Stevia to taste

117 calories

Pour soya into blender
Add blueberries
Slice and add banana
Put in vanilla essence and add stevia to taste
Whizz until blended

Not just one, but two, superfoods – blueberries and bananas- in this!

Vanilla, Celery and Blueberry Fix

180ml (6 fl.oz) vanilla soya milk
1 celery stalk
84g (3 oz) blueberries
Stevia
Ice

120 calories

Pour soya into blender
Chop celery and place in blender
Add blueberries and ice
Blitz completely

As well as lowering blood pressure, celery has cancer preventing properties

Banana and Strawberry Kiss

2 tablespoons fat-free natural yoghurt
1 small banana
56g (2oz) frozen strawberries
150ml (5 fl.oz) almond milk
Stevia to taste

121 calories

Spoon yoghurt into blender
Slice and add in the banana
Add the strawberries
Pour in almond milk
Blend at the highest speed setting

*Banana thickens and strawberries colour this creamy
smoothie*

Spicy Surprise

56g (2 oz) frozen blueberries
1 teaspoon cocoa powder
1 very small banana
14g (½ oz) baby spinach
Small pinch cayenne pepper
1 teaspoon honey
240ml (8 fl.oz) water

121 calories

Put blueberries into blender
Add cocoa powder
Chop and add banana
Put in spinach
Sprinkle on pepper
Add honey
Pour in water
Blitz until smooth

*The flavonoids in cocoa increase the flow of blood and
oxygen to the brain*

Strawberry Crush

120ml (4 fl.oz) fat-free natural yoghurt
60ml (2 fl.oz) skimmed milk
112g (4oz) strawberries, fresh or frozen

122 calories

Put yoghurt into blender
Pour in milk
Add strawberries
Whizz thoroughly

Some say strawberries can prevent wrinkles; I say,
whether it's true or not they taste delicious!

Peachberry Quencher

60ml (2 fl.oz) apple juice
4 tablespoons fat-free vanilla yogurt
84ml (3 oz) frozen peach slices
56g (2 oz) frozen raspberries
180ml (6 fl.oz) water

125 calories

Pour apple juice into blender
Spoon in yoghurt
Add frozen peach slices
Add raspberries
Pour in water
Blend completely

Unsurprisingly, yoghurt is high up in the list of foods that are good for your health – it contains intestine-friendly bacterial cultures that keep your colon healthy.

Melony Green Tea Drink

227g (8 oz) honeydew melon
1 kiwi fruit
120ml (4 fl.oz) water
2 tsp. chopped fresh mint
½ tsp. matcha
Stevia to taste

127 calories

Cut melon into small pieces and place in blender
Halve kiwi fruit, scoop out flesh and add to blender
Pour in water
Add mint and matcha
Blend thoroughly
Add stevia to taste

Matcha green tea is a Japanese tea that comes in powder form. Studies have shown that drinking green tea can significantly lower our risk of developing brain diseases such as Alzheimer's

Peach and Ginger

120ml (4 fl.oz) rice milk
168g (6 oz) frozen peach slices
¼ teaspoon ground ginger
Ice cubes

128 calories

Pour rice milk into blender
Add peach slices and ginger
Pop in ice cubes
Whizz thoroughly

*Rice milk is made from partially milled rice and water
and is good for anyone who is lactose intolerant*

Sweet Banana Smile

150ml (5 fl.oz) skimmed milk
½ medium banana
2 tablespoons low fat natural yoghurt
1 teaspoon clear honey
¼ teaspoon vanilla essence

128 calories

Pour milk into blender
Slice banana and add to milk
Put in yoghurt
Add honey and vanilla essence
Blend thoroughly

Honey has powerful anti bacterial properties

Banana Spice

1 medium banana
¼ teaspoon ground nutmeg
¼ teaspoon ground cinnamon
¼ teaspoon ground cloves
180ml (6 fl.oz) almond milk
Ice

129 calories

Slice banana and put into blender
Add nutmeg, cinnamon and cloves
Pour in almond milk
Add ice
Blitz until smooth

*Nutmeg is purported to be a brain stimulant, cinnamon to
regulate blood sugar and cloves contain healthy
antioxidants*

Sunny Shake

1 small tomato
56g (2 oz) pineapple pieces
112g (4 oz) frozen mango
120ml (4 fl.oz) almond milk

132 calories

Halve tomato and place in blender
Add pineapple
Put in mango
Pour in almond milk
Blend thoroughly

Tomatoes are high in lycopene which is said to be a good preventative for cancer

Smooth Citrus and Strawberry

120ml (4 fl.oz) fat-free vanilla yogurt
60ml (2 fl.oz) cup orange juice
112g (4 oz) strawberries
2 teaspoons lemon juice
¼ teaspoons lemon zest
Crushed ice

132 calories

Spoon yoghurt into blender
Pour in orange juice
Halve and add strawberries
Add lemon juice and zest
Blend until smooth
Pour over crushed ice and stir

Citrus fruits are high in both vitamin C and fibre

Greenie & Creamie

28g (1 oz) pre-packed baby spinach
168g (6 oz) seedless green grapes
60ml (2 fl.oz) coconut water
Ice as desired

139 calories

Put spinach and grapes into blender
Pour in coconut water
Add ice as desired
Blend until totally smooth

*Coconut water is the liquid found inside a coconut. It is
rich in potassium, which helps the body to absorb water
and also to maintain normal blood pressure*

Berry Smooth Banana and Broccoli

5 tablespoons natural yoghurt
70g (2½ oz) frozen mixed berries
28g (1 oz) broccoli
60ml (2 fl.oz) skimmed milk
1 small banana

142 calories

Spoon yoghurt into blender
Add mixed berries
Put in broccoli
Pour in milk
Slice and add banana
Blend until completely smooth

Broccoli contains vitamin A, which is essential for healthy eyesight

Cherrynilla

4 tablespoons fat-free vanilla yoghurt
112g (4 oz) of frozen cherries
120ml (4 fl.oz) cranberry juice

144 calories

Spoon yoghurt into blender
Add cherries
Pour in cranberry juice
Whizz until smooth

Cherries reduce inflammation, are a natural painkiller and improve the quality of your sleep – but best without the stones which can damage your teeth and mess up your blender!

Cinnamon Spiced Berries

56g (2 oz) blackberries
56g (2 oz) strawberries
56g (2 oz) blueberries
120ml (4 fl.oz) soya milk
Pinch ground cinnamon
Stevia to taste
Ice cubes

149 calories

Cut strawberries in half
Put all berries into blender
Pour in soya milk
Add cinnamon, stevia and ice cubes
Blend until smooth

It is said that cinnamon can boost memory. It certainly has a memorable smell

Carribean Sunset

1 small papaya
1 peach
1 passion fruit
180ml (6 fl oz) coconut water
Crushed ice

149 calories

Peel and deseed papaya and put flesh into blender
Slice and add peach
Slice open passion fruit and scoop flesh with seeds into
blender
Pour in coconut water
Blend thoroughly, pour over crushed ice and serve

*The seeds in passion fruit are good for you as they
contain lots of fibre which is important for you because it
keeps your large intestine cleaned out and keeps you
regular (the seeds are crunchy too!)*

Spinach and Melon

75ml (2½ fl.oz) fat-free vanilla yoghurt
56g (2 oz) baby spinach leaves
336g (12 oz) honeydew melon
Ice

150 calories

Spoon yoghurt into blender
Tear and add spinach leaves
Chop melon into small chunks and add
Put in a few ice cubes
Whizz until smooth

*Honeydew melons are good for maintaining healthy skin,
hair, and keeping your weight down*

Spiced Carrot, Apple and Orange

120ml (4 fl.oz) carrot juice
½ green apple
1 teaspoons freshly grated ginger
120ml (4 fl.oz) freshly squeezed orange juice
Ice cubes

150 calories

Pour carrot juice into blender
Core, chop and add apple
Add grated ginger
Pour in orange juice
Pop in ice cubes
Blitz until blended

Ginger is a well known cure for nausea and travel sickness; it's antibacterial and excellent for your digestive tract

Quirky Carrot with Apple

120ml (4 fl.oz) carrot juice
60ml (2 fl.oz) apple juice
60ml (2 fl.oz) fat-free natural yoghurt
½ eating apple
¼ teaspoon cinnamon powder
Ice cubes

152 calories

Pour Carrot and apple juices into blender
Spoon in yoghurt
Core, chop and add apple
Sprinkle with cinnamon
Add ice cubes
Blitz until smooth

*Apple is good for your skin except when it's thrown at
you!*

Orange and Yoghurt Paradise

240ml (8 fl.oz) orange juice with bits
4 tablespoons fat-free yoghurt
¼ teaspoon vanilla essence
A few ice cubes

153 calories

Pour orange juice into blender
Spoon in yoghurt
Add vanilla essence and ice cubes
Whizz until blended

*Oranges are tangy, sweet and a brilliant source of
vitamin C*

Funky Melon

1 tablespoon of ground flax seed
60ml (2 fl.oz) skimmed milk
112g (4 oz) watermelon
1 nectarine
Ice

154 calories

Put flax seed into blender
Pour in milk
Deseed watermelon and add flesh to blender
Slice and add nectarine
Add ice and whizz on high setting to blend

*The mildly nutty flavour of the flax seeds goes well with
the fruit and the fibre in it fills you up nicely*

Veggies and Fruits

28g (1 oz) kale leaves without ribs and stems
120ml (4 fl.oz) apple juice
1 small stalk celery
1 small banana
tablespoon fresh lemon juice
60ml (2 fl.oz) water
Ice cubes

156 calories

Shred the kale leaves and put into blender
Pour in apple juice
Chop and add celery and banana
Pour in lemon juice, water and ice cubes
Whizz until smooth

*Kale is a wonderfully healthy vegetable packed with
calcium, soluble fibre, antioxidants and vitamins*

Vital Vitamin Booster

60ml (2 fl.oz) orange juice
56g (2 oz) frozen blackberries
1small kiwi fruit
1 small apricot
60ml (2 fl.oz) prune juice
Ice

158 calories

Pour orange juice into blender
Add blackberries
Halve kiwi fruit, scoop out flesh and put in blender
Chop and add apricot flesh
Pour in prune juice
Add ice
Combine all ingredients on a high setting

All the goodness of vitamins and a small measure of
prune juice to keep you regular!

Breezy Berry and Green Tea

120ml (4 fl.oz) orange juice
120ml (4 fl.oz) green tea
112g (4 oz) frozen mixed berries
1 small banana
Handful of fresh spinach

159 calories

Pour orange juice and green tea into blender
Add mixed berries
Slice and add banana
Put in spinach
Blend until smooth

*Green tea has many health benefits one of which is,
reportedly, preventing hair loss.*

Fruity Treat

56g (2 oz) strawberries
112g (4 oz) fresh or canned pineapple
150ml (5 fl.oz) orange juice
Crushed ice

161 calories

Put strawberries into blender
Add pineapple, cut into chunks if necessary
Pour in orange juice
Whizz thoroughly in blender
Pour into glass over crushed ice

A good dose of vitamin C in this serving

Berrylumptious

120ml (4 fl.oz) skimmed milk
56g (2 oz) frozen mixed berries
180ml (6 fl.oz) orange juice

162 calories

Pour milk into blender
Add mixed berries
Pour in orange juice
Blend completely

Berries contain antioxidants to fight the free radicals in our bodies which cause ageing and affect our health adversely

Banalmondilla

240ml (8 fl.oz) skimmed milk
1 small banana
¼ teaspoon vanilla essence
Couple of drops almond extract
Pinch ground cinnamon

162 calories

Pour milk into blender
Slice and add banana
Add vanilla essence and almond extract
Blend and serve sprinkled with cinnamon

Skimmed milk is kind to your waistline

Ginger Perk

60ml (2 fl.oz) pineapple juice
120ml (4 fl.oz) orange juice
1 small banana
½ teaspoon grated ginger root
Ice cubes

167 calories

Pour pineapple juice and orange juice into blender
Chop and add banana
Put in grated ginger and ice cubes
Blend on high setting

*Among its many medicinal properties ginger is known for
its antifungal, antibacterial and antiviral benefits. Has to
be good for you then!*

Tastebud Tantaliser

168g (6 oz) honeydew melon
4 tablespoons fat-free lemon yogurt
84g (3 oz) seedless green grapes
2 teaspoons fresh mint
Crushed ice

169 calories

Dice melon and put into blender
Spoon in yoghurt
Add grapes
Chop and add mint
Whizz until smooth and pour onto crushed ice
Stir well and serve

Pterostilbene, which is found in green grapes is thought to help prevent cancer and also lower cholesterol levels in the body. It is, however, rather hard to pronounce!

Carrotty Orange

2 medium sized carrots
240ml (8 fl.oz) orange juice with bits
Ice

170 calories

Peel and chop carrots and put into blender
Add orange juice
Blend on high setting until smooth
Add ice and blend again

*Loads of vitamin C in one glass. This vitamin is an
antioxidant that helps us to keep healthy and prevents
damage to the cells in our bodies*

Melon Refresher

168g (6 oz) cantaloupe melon
84g (3 oz) honeydew melon
84g (3 oz) watermelon
60ml (2 fl.oz) mango juice
1 teaspoon lime juice
1 teaspoons honey
5 fresh mint leaves
Ice cubes

170 calories

Dice cantaloupe and honeydew melon
Deseed and dice watermelon
Put all melon chunks into blender
Pour in mango and lime juices
Add honey, mint leaves and ice cubes
Blend until completely smooth

You can freeze puréed watermelon in ice cube trays to chill drinks and add a subtle touch of flavour.

Pineapple Pick-Me Up

112g (4oz) canned pineapple
56g (2 oz) strawberries
150ml (5 fl.oz) pineapple juice
Ice

171 calories

If using pineapple rings, cut into chunks and place in
blender
Add strawberries
Pour in pineapple juice
Blend thoroughly

*The nutrients in this cooling drink provide you with
natural energy*

Berrinilla

120ml (4 fl.oz) fat-free vanilla yogurt
60ml (2 fl.oz) skimmed milk
84g (3 oz) frozen cherries
84g (3 oz) frozen raspberries
Couple of drops vanilla extract
60ml (2 fl.oz) water

172 calories

Put yoghurt into blender
Pour in milk
Add fruit
Drop in vanilla extract
Add water
Blend on high setting until smooth

*The humble raspberry has a high level of antioxidants
which prevent deterioration of your eyes*

Purple Sunset

4 tablespoons low fat vanilla yogurt
1 small peach or 112g (4 oz) frozen peach slices
1 small banana
56g (2 oz) blueberries

172 calories

Put yoghurt into blender
Slice peach and add to blender
Chop banana and add
Put in blueberries
Whizz until smooth

*Research suggests that the chlorogenic acid in
blueberries helps to lower blood sugar levels*

Creamy Fruit Teaser

3 tablespoons low fat natural yoghurt
112g (4 oz) pineapple chunks
42g (1½ oz) frozen peach slices
56g (2 oz) blueberries
60ml (2 fl.oz) pineapple juice

175 calories

Spoon yoghurt into blender
Put in pineapple chunks
Add peach slices
Add blueberries
Pour in pineapple juice
Blend until creamy and smooth

Plenty of health-giving antioxidants in these blueberries

Spicy Pumpkin

7 tablespoons pumpkin puree
120ml (4 fl.oz) water
120ml (4 fl.oz) skimmed milk
1 tablespoon clear honey
pinch of ground nutmeg
Ice

175 calories

Spoon puree into blender
Pour in water and milk
Add honey, nutmeg and ice
Blend briefly until smooth

*Zinc and alphahydroxy-acids in pumpkins are thought to
help reduce signs of aging*

Smooth Slimmer

1 small banana
120ml (4 fl.oz) orange juice
120ml (4 fl.oz) skimmed milk

176 calories

Slice banana and put into blender
Pour in orange juice and skimmed milk
Blend thoroughly

Bananas contain important amino acids that our bodies need

Green Tonic

½ avocado
Juice of 1 lime
Handful baby spinach
240ml (8 fl.oz) water

176 calories

Pour water into blender
Scoop flesh from avocado and add carefully to water (to avoid splashing)
Squeeze lime and add juice to blender
Put in spinach
Combine until smooth

Spinach is rich in iron and helps prevent anaemia

Ripe and Rosy Rollover

60ml (2 fl.oz) vanilla yoghurt
56g (2 oz) fresh ripe rhubarb
1 small banana
120 ml (4 fl.oz) cranberry juice

176 calories

Spoon yoghurt into blender
Chop and add rhubarb
Slice and add banana
Pour in cranberry juice
Whizz well until smooth

Cranberry is great for the kidneys and urinary tract

Berry and Citrus

56g (2 oz) blueberries
120ml (4 fl.oz) orange juice
½ tangerine
½ orange
½ grapefruit
Ice cubes

177 calories

Put blueberries into blender
Pour in orange juice
Add segments of citrus fruits
Pop in ice cubes
Whizz until smooth

*Low in calories but high in vitamins, grapefruit is an ideal weight loss fruit. Some people, though, are on medications like statins, that clash with it. If you are one of those, use **1½ tangerines** instead to keep the calorie count for this smoothie*

Peachy Mango Temptation

112g (4 oz) frozen peach slices
112g (4 oz) frozen mango chunks
120ml (4 fl.oz) peach nectar
1 tablespoon lime juice

184 calories

Place peach slices in blender
Add mango chunks
Pour in peach nectar
Add lime juice
Whizz in blender until smooth

Peaches are low in calories with lots of healthy minerals and vitamins

Merry Berry Cherry

120ml (4 fl.oz) fat-free natural yoghurt
112g (4 oz) strawberries
112g (4 oz) frozen cherries
2 tsp. ground flax seed
¾ tsp. pure vanilla extract

185 calories

Spoon yoghurt into blender
Halve and add strawberries
Put in cherries
Add flax seed and vanilla extract
Blend on high setting

*Cherries contain anthocyanins: natural pigments said to
help to prevent cancer. Cherries taste good too!*

Raspberry and Peach Delight

112g (4 oz) peach yoghurt
112g (4 oz) frozen raspberries
180 ml (6 fl.oz) orange juice

188 calories

Spoon yoghurt into blender
Add raspberries
Pour in orange juice
Blend thoroughly

Raspberries are very good for cleansing your gut!

Lemony Apricot & Mango

180ml (6 fl.oz) skimmed milk
3 apricots
112g (4 oz) frozen mango slices
2 tablespoons lemon juice
¼ teaspoon vanilla essence
Ice cubes

193 calories

Pour milk into blender
Slice apricots
Add apricots to blender
Add in mango slices
Pour in lemon juice, vanilla essence and ice cubes
Blend until smooth and creamy

*Apricots, whilst low in calories, are high in dietary fibre,
vitamins and minerals*

Spicy Almond with Kale

1 small banana
56g (2 oz) kale, stems removed
180ml (6 fl.oz) almond milk
¾ tablespoon almond butter
pinch each of ground cinnamon, nutmeg and ginger.

194 calories

Slice banana before placing in blender
Chop and add kale
Pour in almond milk
Add almond butter
Put in spices
Blend until completely smooth

*Almond milk is thought to help reduce the risk of
Alzheimers and osteoporosis, because it contains lots of
vitamin D which helps in cell building*

Fruity Oaty Shake

180ml (6 fl.oz) fat-free natural yoghurt
112g (4 oz) frozen raspberries
60ml (2 fl.oz) skimmed milk
1 tablespoon oatmeal
60ml (2 fl.oz) water

196 calories

Spoon yoghurt into blender
Add raspberries
Pour in milk
Add oatmeal
Pour in water
Blend everything thoroughly

Oats are an excellent source of many healthy nutrients, two of which are magnesium and protein. Magnesium is said to combat stress and protein is essential for energy and to rebuild tissue body tissue

Tasty Tummy Soother

120ml (4 fl.oz) fat-free natural yoghurt
56g (2oz) papaya
56g (2 oz) frozen sliced peaches
1 small pear
1 teaspoon ground flax seed
½ tsp ground ginger
2 mint leaves

204 calories

Spoon yoghurt into blender
Peel, deseed and cube papaya
Add peaches and papaya to yoghurt
Peel, chop and add pear
Put in flax seed and ginger
Blend thoroughly and garnish with mint leaves

Among its many health benefits papaya relieves digestion problems, improves your skin and protects your heart and eyes

Peanut Butter Creamer

4 tablespoons fat-free vanilla yogurt
120ml (4 fl.oz) pineapple juice
1 tablespoon of smooth peanut butter
120ml (4 fl.oz) almond milk
Ice

206 calories

Spoon yoghurt into blender
Pour in pineapple juice
Add peanut butter
Pour in almond milk
Pop in ice
Blend thoroughly

*Americans eat enough peanut butter each year to cover
the floor of the Grand Canyon, but there's still enough
left for your smoothie wherever you live!*

Blueberry Orange

4 tablespoons fat-free vanilla yoghurt
112g (4 oz) blueberries
120ml (4 fl.oz) orange juice
120ml (4 fl.oz) skimmed milk
½ teaspoon vanilla essence

206 calories

Spoon yoghurt into blender
Add blueberries
Pour in orange juice and milk
Add vanilla essence
Blend until completely smooth

*With superstar blueberries, vitamin C rich orange juice
and bone-healthy calcium in the milk, it's a truly health-
giving drink*

Spicy Nutty Pear, Orange and Rocket

120ml (4 fl.oz) natural fat-free yogurt
1 teaspoon of ground ginger
1small ripe pear
1 tablespoon chopped walnuts
84g (3 oz) rocket (arugula)
120ml (4 fl.oz) almond milk
Ice cubes

211 calories

Spoon yoghurt into blender
Add ginger
Core, chop and add pear
Add walnuts and rocket
Pour in almond milk
Pop in ice cubes
Blend completely

*Walnuts contain vitamins, minerals and antioxidants and
also help to give you energy*

Pear, Peach and Strawberry

4 tablespoons fat-free natural yoghurt
1 small soft pear
1 small ripe peach
112g (4 oz) strawberries
120ml (4 fl.oz) coconut water

216 calories

Spoon yoghurt into blender
Peel and slice pear and peach before adding to blender
Halve and add strawberries
Pour in coconut water
Whizz on high setting until well combined

For a mild laxative look no further than pears. It's the pectin in them that has this effect on the body

Grapefully Smoothful

112g (4 oz) green seedless grapes
120ml (4 fl.oz) grape juice
84g (3 oz) frozen blueberries
75 ml (2½ fl.oz) almond milk

217 calories

Put grapes into blender
Pour in grape juice
Add blueberries
Pour in almond milk
Whizz thoroughly

Grapes are good for the heart. They raise nitric oxide levels in the blood which helps to prevent blood clots and staves off heart attacks and strokes.

Strawberry-Kiwi Fantasia

210ml (7 fl.oz) apple juice
1 small banana
1 kiwi fruit
56g (2 oz) frozen strawberries

223 calories

Pour apple juice into blender
Chop and add banana
Halve kiwi fruit, scoop out flesh and put in blender
Add strawberries
Blend thoroughly

Give your immune system a helping hand with all this vitamin C

Pomegranate surprise

1 small banana
1 kiwi fruit
70g (2½ oz) blueberries
56g (2 oz) strawberries
90ml (3 fl.oz) pomegranate juice

224 calories

Slice banana and put into blender
Halve kiwi and scoop flesh into blender
Add blueberries
Halve strawberries and add
Pour in pomegranate juice
Whizz until smooth

Pomegranate juice is a tasty way to settle stomach upsets

Berry Beetroot

4 tablespoons fat-free natural yoghurt
168g (6 oz) blueberries
84g (3 oz) frozen raspberries
56g (2 oz) cooked beetroot
60ml (2 fl.oz) orange juice
Stevia

227 calories

Spoon yoghurt into blender
Put in blueberries
Add raspberries
Peel, slice and add beetroot
Pour in orange juice
Add stevia if sweeter taste is required
Blend everything

The beta cyanin in beetroot helps detoxify your liver

Blueberry and Bananalicous

150ml (5 fl oz) apple juice
120ml (4 fl.oz) natural yoghurt
1 small banana
112g (4 oz) blueberries

229 calories

Pour apple juice into blender
Spoon in yoghurt
Chop and add banana
Put in blueberries
Combine until smooth

*There is exciting new research suggesting that regular
consumption of blueberries may not only be beneficial
for improving memory but might also slow down, or
postpone, various cognitive problems associated with
aging*

Berrylicious Banana

60ml (2 fl.oz) soya milk
1 small ripe banana
1 tablespoon smooth peanut butter
168g (6 oz) raspberries
Crushed ice

230 calories

Pour soya milk into blender
Slice and add banana
Put in peanut butter
Add raspberries and ice
Blend to a smooth consistency

Peanut butter contains resveratrol -an antioxidant which,
it is thought, helps prevent heart disease and cancer

Smoothberry and Beetroot

1 teaspoon honey
60ml (2 fl.oz) low-fat natural yoghurt
112g (4 oz) raw beetroot
2 tablespoons granola
168g (6 oz) mixed blueberries
120ml (4 fl.oz) freshly squeezed orange juice
Ice cubes

230 calories

Spoon honey and yoghurt into blender
Peel, finely chop and add beetroot
Add granola and blueberries
Pour in orange juice
Pop in ice
Blend on high setting until completely smooth

Betaine in beetroot may help to cheer you up because it increases serotonin, a mood enhancer which is naturally produced in the body

Minty Avocado, Lime and Mango

½ small avocado
168g (6 oz) frozen mango slices
1 tablespoon lime juice
1 tablespoon chopped fresh mint
Stevia
240ml (8 fl.oz) water

234 calories

Scoop flesh of avocado into blender
Add mango slices
Pour in lime juice
Add chopped mint
Put in stevia to taste
Pour in water
Blend thoroughly

*The avocado is believed to have originated in Mexico,
where the name comes from an Aztec word: 'ahuacatl'
meaning 'testicle' which refers to the fruit's shape (just
thought you'd like to know that!)*

Pear, Peach and Cinnamon

120ml (4 fl.oz) apple juice
120ml (4 fl.oz) fat-free natural yoghurt
1 small ripe pear
84g (3 oz) frozen peach slices
½ teaspoon cinnamon

238 calories

Pour apple juice into blender
Spoon in yoghurt
Core, chop and add pear
Add peach slices
Sprinkle with cinnamon
Whizz until completely combined

Pears boost your immune system, help prevent osteoporosis, increase energy and aid your digestion – in short- they're very good for you!

Mildly Nutty and Fruity

1 tablespoon ground flax seed
4 tablespoons fat-free natural yoghurt.
120ml (4 fl.oz) pineapple juice
1 kiwi fruit
½ papaya
84g (3 oz) frozen mango slices

246 calories

Put flax seed and yoghurt into blender
Pour in pineapple juice
Halve kiwi fruit, scoop out flesh and add
Deseed, peel, chop and add papaya
Add mango slices
Blitz until smooth

Low in calories, ground flaxseed provides you with
essential vitamins and minerals in this delicious smoothie

Reference Pages:
Calorie Counter, Calorie Chart, Indexes

Your Calorie Counter

Here, foods are grouped according to their calorie content to enable you to pick, choose and substitute according to your personal preferences. It is followed by a more detailed chart arranged in alphabetical order for ease of reference.

0 – 10 Calories

Vegetables

Mint leaves (**0**)
Chives, 1 tsp chopped (**1**)
Mixed herbs, dried, 1 pinch (**1**)
Onion, 1 tsp raw chopped (**4**)
Mushrooms, 28g (1 oz) (**4**)
Parsley, 10 sprigs (**5**)
Cucumber, 6 slices (**5**)
Celery, 1 stick (**5**)
Garlic, 1 clove (**5**)
Radishes, 4 (**5**)
Iceberg lettuce, 84g (**5**)
Spring onions, 6 (**5**)
Leaf lettuce 84g (**5**)

Drinks
Black tea (**0**)
Earl Grey tea (**0**)
Green tea (**0**)
Rooibos Tea (0)
Diet cola (**0**)

Twinings infusions (**2**)
Coffee, filtered, black (**1**)
Tea w/skimmed milk (**10**)
 Bovril (beef extract), 1 tsp (**10**)
 Marmite, 1 tsp (**10**)

Miscellaneous

Salt (**0**)
Vinegar (**0**)
Stevia extract (sweetener) (**0**)
Mustard 1 tsp (**5**)

11 – 20 Calories

Vegetables

Cabbage, 112g (**15**)
Asparagus, 4 spears (**15**)
Courgette (zucchini), 1 small (**15**)
Onion, 1 small (**20**)
Cherry tomatoes, 6 (**20**)
Sweet Pepper, 1 any colour (**20**)

Fruit

Plum, 1 medium (**30**)
Lemon, 1 medium (**15**)
Apricot 1 (**15**)
Satsuma 1 (**20**)

Dairy

Cheese triangle, extra light (**20**)

Drinks

Almond milk 120ml (**12**)

Tea w/ semi-skimmed milk (**15**)
Tea w/ whole milk (**20**)

Miscellaneous

Sauce, brown, 1 tbsp (**13**)
Ketchup, 1 tbsp (**15**)
Honey, 1 tsp (**20**)
Ryvita Original, 1 crispbread (**20**)

21 – 30 Calories

Vegetables

Tomato, 1 medium (**25**)
Carrot, 1 medium (**25**)
Beet, 2 small whole cooked (**30**)
Cauliflower, dry, 84g (**30**)

Fruit

Blueberries, 50g (**25**)
Melon, Honeydew 100g (**30**)

Dairy

Olive spread, 1 tsp (**25**)
Parmesan cheese, grated 1 tbsp (**25**)

Miscellaneous

Sugar, white, 1 tsp (**25**)
Rice cakes, 1 (**30**)
Peanut butter, 1 tsp (**30**)

31 – 40 Calories

Meat / Fish

Ham, sliced pre-packed 1 medium slice (**35**)

Vegetables

Onion, sliced, 168g (**40**)
Trimmed cut green beans, 168g (**40**)

Fruit

Pineapple, canned in juice, 1 ring (**35**)
Grapes, 10 (**35**)
Plum, 1 large (**35**)
Peach, 1 small fresh (**35**)
Tangerine, 1 small (**35**)
Grapefruit, half (**40**)
Apricots, canned in juice, 3 halves (**40**)

Dairy

Butter / margarine, 1 pat (**35**)
Extra Light Philadelphia soft cheese, 35g mini tub (**38**)

Drinks
Soya milk light, 120ml (**35**)
Options low fat chocolate drink, 1 serving (**40**)
Tomato juice, 120ml (**40**)

Miscellaneous

Cream crackers, low fat, 2 (**35**)
Marmalade / Jam, 1 tsp (**40**)

41 – 50 Calories

Vegetables

Broccoli, 112g **(45)**
Carrots, grated 112g **(45)**
Beet, cooked & diced, 168g **(50)**
Tomatoes, canned, chopped, 168g **(50)**

Fruit

Watermelon cubed, 168g **(45)**
Kiwi Fruit, 1 **(45)**
Strawberries, 168g **(45)**
Cherries, 10 **(50)**
Pear, 1 medium **(50)**

Drinks

Spring vegetable cup soup, 13g sachet **(45)**

51 – 100 Calories

Meat / Fish

Fish finger, grilled 1 **(55)**
Prawns, boiled 20 **(60)**
Back bacon, lean, 1 rasher **(65)**
Quorn vegetarian sausage, 1 **(70)**
Chicken drumstick, skinless, cooked, 1 **(75)**
Sole, baked, 84g **(80)**
Quorn vegetarian burger, 1 **(80)**
Rollmop herring, 1 **(90)**
Linda McCartney vegetarian sausage, 1 **(95)**

Vegetables

Peas, cooked from frozen, 168g (**65**)
Carrots, cooked, 168g (**70**)
New potatoes, boiled, 100g (**75**)
Potato waffle, 1 (56g) (**95**)
Corn on the cob, 1 medium (**100**)

Fruit

Apple, 1 small (**55**)
Orange, 1 medium (**60**)
Apples, peeled & sliced, 168g (**65**)
Raspberries, 168g (**65**)
Banana, 1 extra small (less than 6') (**70**)
Sunmaid raisins, 1 small packet (28g) (**92**)

Dairy

Egg, 1 small (**55**)
Egg, 1 medium (**65**)
Egg, 1 large (**75**)
Yoghurt, low fat plain, 125g pot (**80**)
Milk, skimmed, 240ml (**85**)
Egg, 1 large, scrambled or omelette (**100**)

Cereals

Weetabix, 1 biscuit (**65**)
All-Bran cereal, 84g (**80**)
Grape Nuts cereal, 28g (**100**)
Shredded Wheat, 28g (**100**)

Drinks

Leek & Potato cup soup, low fat, 1 sachet (**55**)
Soya milk, 100ml (**55**)
Ovaltine light, 20g serving (**72**)
Red wine, 100ml (**75**)

Chicken noodle soup, canned, 240ml (**75**)
Milk, skimmed, 120ml (**85**)
Grapefruit juice, 240ml (**95**)
Orange juice, 120ml (**100**)

Miscellaneous

Lemon juice, 240ml (**60**)
Honey, 1 tbsp (**65**)
Wholemeal bread, 1 medium slice (**75**)
Crumpet, 1 (**90**)
Peanut butter 1 tbsp (**95**)
Almonds, 14 (**100**)

101 – 200

Meat /Fish

Quorn garlic & parsley sausage, 1 (**104**)
Quorn vegetarian British sausage, 1 (**111**)
Smoked haddock, 100g baked (**115**)
Ham, cooked & sliced, pre-packed 100g (**115**)
Turkey, roast, 84g (**130**)
Roast beef, lean, 70g (**130**)
Tuna, canned in water, 84g (**135**)
Lamb leg, lean roasted, 70g (**135**)
Salmon steak, baked, 84g (**140**)
Halibut, grilled w/ butter, 84g (**140**)
Chicken breast, roasted, 84g (**140**)
Sardines in tomato sauce, 120g can (**148**)
Salmon, smoked, 84g (**150**)
Sirloin steak, lean, grilled 100g (**185**)
Chicken breast, skinless, 130g, grilled (**190**)
Lamb's liver, fried, 84g (**190**)
Quorn Cottage Pie, chilled, prepacked meal, 300g (**200**)

Vegetables

Parsnips, cooked, 168g **(125)**
Potato, baked w/skin, 170g **(160)**
Baked beans, half can **(195)**
Potato, mashed w/skimmed milk, 168g **(200)**

Fruit

Banana, 1 medium **(105)**
Apple, 1 large **(110)**
Dried prunes, 5 large **(115)**

Dairy

Cheddar cheese, grated, 28g **(110)**
Milk, semi-skimmed, 240ml **(120)**
Yoghurt, low fat, flavoured, 125g pot **(125)**
Milk, whole, 240ml **(150)**

Cereals

Rice Crispies, 28g **(110)**
Corn flakes, 28g **(110)**
Muesli original, 45g **(170)**

Drinks

Milk, semi-skimmed, 240ml **(120)**
Milk, whole, 240ml **(150)**
Chicken soup, cream of, canned, 240ml **(190)**

Miscellaneous

Tomato puree, canned, 240ml **(105)**
Macaroni, cooked, 168g (from 84g dry) **(115)**
Olive oil/vegetable oils, 1tbsp **(125)**
Muffin, 1 **(140)**

Peanuts, oil roasted, 28g **(150)**
Cashew nuts, dry roasted, 28g **(165)**
Penne pasta, 50g (dry weight) **(175)**
Split pea soup, condensed, 120ml + water **(180)**
Brazil nuts, 28g **(185)**
Brown rice, long grain, 50g (dry weight) **(185)**
Bagel, 1 **(200)**

Over 200 Calories

Vegetarian Options

Moroccan Tagine ready meal (Easy Bean) **(211 cal)**
Quorn Cottage Pie, ready-meal 300g **(213)**
Nut cutlet, Tesco **(240)**
Cheese & onion crispbake, 1 - Asda (Walmart) **(289 cal)**

Alphabetical Calorie Chart

This chart is designed for ease of reference. Foods and ingredients are given calorie content in the most common measuring units.

Ingredient	Item	28g (1 oz)	30ml (1 fl.oz)	1 Teaspoon	1 Tablespoon
All-Bran cereal		27			
Almond butter		177		34	101
Almond extract				11	
Almond milk, unsweetened			3		
Almonds, 14	100				
Apple, large	110				
Apple, medium	80	15			
Apple, small	55				
Apple juice			15		
Apricots, canned		14			
Apricot, fresh	15				
Asparagus spear	4				
Avocado	322	50			
Bacon, back, lean, rasher	65				
Bagel	200				
Baked beans		20			
Banana, medium	105	25			
Banana, small	70	25			
Brazil nuts		185			
Beans, green trimmed, cut		7			
Beef, roast, lean		52			
Beet leaves	7	8			

Ingredient	Item	28g (1 oz)	30ml (1 fl.oz)	1 Teaspoon	1 Tablespoon
Beetroot, cooked		12			
Beetroot, raw		12			
Berries, mixed		14			
Blackberries		12			
Blueberries		14			
Brazil nuts		185			
Bread, wholemeal, medium, slice	75				
Broccoli		9			
Butter / margarine, 1 pat	35				
Cabbage		4			
Carrot	25	12			
Carrot juice			12		
Cashew nuts, dry roasted		165			
Cauliflower, dry		10			
Cayenne pepper				6	
Celery stalk	5	4			
Cheese, Cheddar, grated,		110			
Cheese triangle, extra light	20				
Cherries, frozen, de-stoned		13			
Cherry	5				
Chicken breast, skinless grilled		41			
Chicken breast, roasted		47			

Ingredient	Item	28g (1 oz)	30ml (1 fl.oz)	1 Teaspoon	1 Tablespoon
Chicken drumstick, skinless, cooked	75				
Chilli sauce, sweet					30
Chives, chopped		8		1	1
Choc drink, Options low fat, serving	40				
Cinnamon, ground				6	
Cloves, ground				6	
Cocoa powder, unsweetened				4	12
Coconut water			6		
Coffee, brewed, black			1		
Coffee, instant granules, black				2	
Cola, diet			0		
Corn flakes		110			
Corn on the cob, medium	100				
Cottage cheese, low fat		30			
Courgette (zucchini), small	15				
Cranberries		13			
Cranberry juice			15		
Cream crackers, low fat, 2	35				
Crumpet	90				
Cucumber, peeled	24	3			
Egg, large	75				
Egg, medium	65				

Ingredient	Item	28g (1 oz)	30ml (1 fl.oz)	1 Teaspoon	1 Tablespoon
Egg, small	55				
Egg noodles, fresh		19			
Falafel		78			
Feta Cheese		74			
Fish finger, grilled	55				
Frankfurter, vegetarian (Tivall)	70				
Fruit infusions (fruit teas), serving	2				
Garlic, 1 clove	5				
Ginger, ground				6	18
Ginger, root		22		2	
Goat's cheese		84			
Granola		95			35
Grape Nuts cereal		100			
Grapefruit	72				
Grapefruit juice			12		
Grape juice			21		
Grapes		20			
Haddock, smoked		32			
Halibut, grilled with butter		47			
Herring, rollmop, 1	90				
Ham, cooked, medium slice	35	32			
Honey				20	60

Ingredient	Item	28g (1 oz)	30ml (1 fl.oz)	1 Teaspoon	1 Tablespoon
Ice		0			
Kale leaves		14			
Ketchup					15
Kiwi fruit	29	13			
Lamb, leg roasted, lean		54			
Lamb's liver, fried		63			
Leek & Potato cup soup, sachet	55				
Lemon without peel	17				
Lemon juice			7		4
Lemon zest				1	
Lettuce, iceberg		1			
Lettuce, leaf		1			
Lime juice			8	1	4
Macaroni, cooked		49			
Mango juice			15		
Marmalade / Jam				40	
Mango pieces, frozen		17			
Melon, cantaloupe		10			
Melon, honeydew		10			
Milk, semi-skimmed			15		
Milk, skimmed			11		
Mint, fresh					1

Ingredient	Item	28g (1 oz)	30ml (1 fl.oz)	1 Teaspoon	1 Tablespoon
Mixed herbs, dried, 1 pinch	1				
Muesli, Alpen original		109			
Muffin	140				
Mushrooms		4			
Mustard				5	
Nectarine	60				
Nut cutlet, Tesco	240				
Nutmeg, ground				12	36
Oatmeal					18
Oats, porridge		112			
Olive spread				25	
Olive oil/vegetable oils					120
Onion, chopped		7		1	4
Onion, small	20				
Orange	62				
Orange, large	86				
Orange juice			15		
Ovaltine light, serving	72				
Papaya, small	59	11			
Parmesan cheese, grated					25
Parsley		10			1
Parsnips, cooked		21			

Ingredient	Item	28g (1 oz)	30ml (1 fl.oz)	1 Teaspoon	1 Tablespoon
Passion fruit	17				
Pasta, (dry weight)		98			
Peach nectar			17		
Peach, small fresh	35				
Peanut butter, smooth				30	90
Peanuts, oil roasted		150			
Pear, Asian medium	50				
Pear, medium	96				
Pear, small	80				
Peas, cooked from frozen		12			
Pepper, ground				5	
Pepper, sweet (bell), any colour	20				
Philadelphia Extra Light, 35g mini tub	38				
Pineapple juice			17		
Pineapple, canned		17			
Pineapple, fresh		14			
Plum, medium	30				
Plum, 1 large	35				
Pomegranate juice			17		
Potato, baked w/skin, 200g	190				
Potato, mashed w/skimmed milk		33			
Potatoes new, boiled		21			

Ingredient	Item	28g (1 oz)	30ml (1 fl.oz)	1 Teaspoon	1 Tablespoon
Prawns, boiled, 20	55				
Prune juice			22		
Prunes, dried, large	23				
Quark		19			15
Quorn Garlic & Parsley Sausage	104				
Quorn Cottage Pie, ready meal, 300g	213				
Quorn Peppered Steak	123				
Quorn Vegetarian Sausage	70				
Quorn Vegetarian Family Roast		30			
Radishes, 4	5				
Raisins, Sunmaid, small packet (28g)	92				
Raspberries		15			
Rhubarb pieces		6			
Rhubarb stalk	11				
Rice cake	30				
Rice milk			15		
Rice, brown long grain, (dry weight)		104			
Rice, white long-grain (cooked weight)		37			
Rice cake	30				
Rice Crispies		110			
Rocket (arugula)		4			

Ingredient	Item	28g (1 oz)	30ml (1 fl.oz)	1 Teaspoon	1 Tablespoon
Salmon, smoked		50			
Salmon steak, baked		47			
Salt		0		0	
Sardines in tomato sauce, 120g can	148				
Satsuma	20				
Sauce, brown					13
Sausage, Linda McCartney Vegetarian	95				
Shredded Wheat, 1 biscuit	75				
Sole, baked		27			
Sorbet, orange		25			
Sour cream				8	24
Soy sauce					9
Soya milk, sweetened			16		
Soya milk, unsweetened			8		
Soya milk, vanilla			14		
Spinach		7			
Spring onions, 6	5				
Spring vegetable cup soup, sachet	45				
Steak, sirloin, lean grilled		52			
Stevia		0		0	0
Strawberries		9			

Ingredient	Item	28g (1 oz)	30ml (1 fl.oz)	1 Teaspoon	1 Tablespoon
Sugar, white				25	
Tabasco sauce				1	
Tangerine	35				
Tea, green, serving	0				
Tea, Earl Grey, serving	0				
Tea, Rooibos, serving	0				
Tea, black, serving	0				
Tea, green, serving	0				
Tea w/skimmed milk, serving	10				
Tea w/ whole milk, serving	20				
Tea w/ semi-skimmed milk	15				
Tofu, ready-marinated		64			
Tofu, smoked (Taifun)		52			
Tomato, medium	25	5			
Tomatoes, cherry, 6	20	5			
Tomato, small	18	5			
Tomato juice			10		
Tomatoes, canned, chopped		8			
Tuna, canned in water		45			
Turkey, roast		43			
Vanilla essence				2	
Vanilla extract				12	

Ingredient	Item	28g (1 oz)	30ml (1 fl.oz)	1 Teaspoon	1 Tablespoon
Vinegar				0	0
Waffle, potato, 56g	95				
Walnuts		194			40
Water		0		0	0
Watercress		4			
Watermelon		9			
Weetabix, biscuit	65				
Yeast extract (Marmite)				10	
Yoghurt, lemon, fat-free		24			12
Yoghurt, natural, fat-free		16			8
Yoghurt, vanilla, fat-free		16			8

Index of Lucy's Recipes

Recipes marked with an asterisk (*) are suitable for vegetarians

	Calories	Page
Courgette and Chive Omelette*	127	92
Salmon and Cream Cheese Toasty Munch	179	94
Potato, Onion & Greens Soup*	112	97
Chicken Liver Lunch	183	100
Greek Salad*	159	102
Tuna Salad	185	105
Hot Toddy*	69	107
Smoked Salmon & Radishes w/ Poppy Seed Dressing	120	110
Cauliflower and Onion Soup*	87	112
Refreshing Raspberry Fizz*	60	115
Minty Pineapple and Grapefruit*	168	118

Dinners

	Calories	Page
Tangy Tomato and Mozzarella Salad*	279	69
Ham & Roasted Vegetables	210	72
Ham, Cheese & Tomato Omelette	250	75
Spicy Chicken with Tomato, Pepper & Mint Salad	215	78
Halibut with Barbecue Sauce	239	81
Spicy Chicken Breast	240	84
Spicy Fish Dish	258	87
Beefy Chilli Stir Fry	227	89
Lemon and Parsley Haddock with Green Beans	200	91
Chilli Chicken Stir Fry	180	93
Vegetable Stir Fry*	191	95
Grilled Lamb Chop Special	270	98
Mediterranean Beef	225	100
Baked Vegetables with Salmon	188	103
Chicken & Mushroom Broth, Thai Style	179	106
Mediterranean Chicken	203	108
Chicken Tandoori	206	110
Courgette, Lentil and Feta Salad*	276	113
Salmon fishcake with Petits Pois	290	116
Vegetable Chilli*	181	118

Index of Emily's Smoothies

Listed in groups according to calorie count, lowest first: same order as the recipes in the text

Berry Smooth Banana and Broccoli
Cherrynilla
Cinnamon Spiced Berries
Carribean Sunset
Spinach and Melon
Spiced Carrot, Apple and Orange

151-200 Calories: Pages 159 - 186

Quirky Carrot with Apple
Orange and Yoghurt Paradise
Funky Melon
Veggies and Fruits
Vital Vitamin Booster
Breezy Berry and Green Tea
Fruity Treat
Berrylumptious
Banalmondilla
Ginger Perk
Tastebud Tantaliser
Carrotty Orange
Melon Refresher
Pineapple Pick-Me Up
Berrinilla
Purple Sunset
Creamy Fruit Teaser
Spicy Pumpkin
Smooth Slimmer
Green Tonic
Ripe and Rosy Rollover
Berry and Citrus
Peachy Mango Temptation
Merry Berry Cherry
Raspberry and Peach Delight
Lemony Apricot & Mango
Spicy Almond with Kale
Fruity Oaty Shake

201-246 Calories: Pages 187 - 201

Tasty Tummy Soother
Peanut Butter Creamer
Blueberry Orange
Spicy Nutty Pear, Orange and Rocket
Pear, Peach and Strawberry
Grapefully Smoothful
Strawberry-Kiwi Fantasia
Pomegranate surprise
Berry Beetroot
Blueberry and Bananalicous
Berrylicious Banana
Smoothberry and Beetroot
Minty Avocado, Lime and Mango
Pear, Peach and Cinnamon
Mildly Nutty and Fruity

www.ingramcontent.com/pod-product-compliance
Lightning Source LLC
Chambersburg PA
CBHW060456290526
45791CB00001B/146